SHADOW OVER MY BRAIN

'In life – there are no solutions – there are forces
on the move, forces one must set in motion, and then
the solutions follow.'

Antoine de Saint-Expurery

SHADOW OVER MY BRAIN

A Battle Against Parkinson's Disease

CECIL TODES

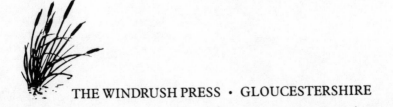

THE WINDRUSH PRESS · GLOUCESTERSHIRE

First published in Great Britain by
The Windrush Press,
Windrush House,
Main Street,
Adlestrop,
Moreton-in-Marsh,
Gloucestershire
1990

British Library Cataloguing in Publication Data
Todes, Cecil
   Shadow over my brain: a battle against Parkinson's disease
   1. Parkinson's Disease victims, – Biographies
   I. Title
   362.1968330092

   ISBN 0-900075-86-4

Typeset by DP Photosetting, Aylesbury, Bucks
Printed and bound in Great Britain by Biddles Ltd, Guildford

To Lili,   who else!

Contents

Foreword

Oliver Sacks

There have been, in the nearly two hundred years since Parkinson's *Essay on the Shaking Palsy*, innumerable 'medical' accounts of Parkinson's disease. There have also been a small number of 'inside narratives' – descriptions of living with Parkinson's disease by patients themselves (those of Ivan Vaughan and Sidney Dorros at once come to mind). But there has never been, to my knowledge, an account which brings both perspectives together – that of the patient *and* that of the doctor. There have, indeed, been physicians with Parkinson's disease (the famous neurologist Henry Head was among them), but none of them, up to now, has given us a personal account of what it is to live with the disease. In this way, as in many others, Dr Todes's account is unique.

Dr Todes was born in South Africa, trained first as a dentist, but then, realizing that his deepest interests lay in human behaviour and relationships, came to England, went to medical school, and then on to psychoanalytic training. It was during this, as a healthy young man in his thirties, that Dr Todes found himself stricken with Parkinson's disease. He fought against the diagnosis – this sentencing, in the prime of life, to a stealthily-disabling chronic neurological disorder: which of us, finding ourselves in such a position, would not? When the diagnosis could no longer be fought, Dr Todes fought – and goes on fighting – with the disease itself; with its peculiar distresses and disabilities; and with the excitements and disappointments, and sometimes bizarre side-effects, of medications. This fighting quality is a great positive in his life; it has enabled him to continue at his daily, taxing explorations of the human psyche, to hold together as a deep and vivid person, and to write a brave (and often funny) and very gripping book.

As a person with Parkinson's disease, Dr Todes has been subjected to, or subjected himself to, innumerable treatments – chemical and otherwise: he has taken (to give an abbreviated list) L-dopa, Sinemet, Madopar, amantadine, bromocriptine, pergolide, lisuride (this last by a subcutaneous pump in Pamplona – a quite horrifying, but in its gruesome way, entertaining episode); he has taken Deprenyl, endorphins, tyrosine, injectable iron, nauseating injections of apomorphine; he has had a whirl with biofeedback, acupuncture, allergic desensitization, spiritualism; and he is one of the very few people in the world to have had living foetal cells transplanted in his brain.

Dr Todes, then, has been through the entire gamut of treatments for Parkinsonism – he describes them all (and his often extravagant hopes and disappointments with them) with vividness and irony; and he describes too a spectrum of doctors, of neurologists, ranging all the way from almost saintly to monstrous – doctors whom he can see, complexly, with a double eye, for he finds himself, in relation to them, at once patient and colleague.

Dr Todes's account of living with Parkinson's disease, coping with it, and of his ups and downs with doctors, is well-told, fast-paced, affecting – and funny. But the special strength of this book, to my mind, lies in its *depth* – its depth of psychiatric and moral insight, its exploration, at the deepest level, of what it means to be Parkinsonian. Parkinson's disease, as is well known, can cause tremor, stiffness, difficulty moving, soft and hurried speech – but it is not a purely motor disorder; there can be a variety of subtle effects on thinking, dreaming, imagery, mood, emotional expression, attitudes, body-image, etc. which have never been adequately described. Dr Todes has been forced, as a sufferer, but one with a very acute and analytic mind, to explore all of these common, but hitherto scarcely-described ramifications of Parkinson's disease, its effects on the psyche, on the whole person, of the sufferer. He speaks here of a 'somatopsychic approach' – and the insights which have been given him by his own illness, and his understanding of it, have led him, as a physician, to pay much more attention to the whole physical and psychic economy of his patients' lives, instead of a narrow, purely physical or purely mental approach.

A very special experience set out in this book and also in the articles which Dr Todes has contributed to the medical literature, stems from the unique exploration which he has made with a number of other highly intelligent, articulate patients with youthful-onset Parkinsonism like himself. When his first symptom (tremor) appeared, Dr Todes wondered if it could be a psychiatric symptom – a masked expression of unconscious needs or conflict, like a hysterical symptom. This is a notion he soon gave up; but he does feel that a pattern of childhood loss and bereavement, and a complex vulnerable state of mind arising from this (which includes elements of depression, but is not simply depressive) may have played a part in *predisposing* him to become Parkinsonian – and he has found similar patterns to the lives of other patients with this youthful-onset Parkinsonism. Whether there is in fact a 'Parkinsonian personality' must be questioned, but its questioning will require the sort of in-depth exploration of young Parkinsonian patients such as Dr Todes himself has pioneered.

Dr Todes tells us the story of a grim disease and a grim struggle, yet it is not grimness which is finally conveyed. One has, rather, a feeling of courage and resource, a feeling of a man not merely coping with, but transcending his condition; and of a man who has been driven to experience life, and think about it, more deeply than most of us do, precisely because he has had to contend with illness. 'I do not say that suffering makes us better,' writes Nietzsche, 'but it makes us more profound.'

Thus the final note of this book – as of all the best books about illness – is not one of defeat, brokenness or lamentation; but rather one of affirmation, and even celebration, at man's capacity to lead the fullest life, to make the most of life, to live creatively, cockily, defiantly, and even triumphantly, even in the face of irremediable adversity. This, after all, is what being human is about.

CHAPTER 1

The Day My Watch Stopped

One day, my watch stopped; it was a Nivada Automatic that my friends had given me for my twenty-first birthday just before I left my home country. I was attached to it and anxious to keep it going, so I packed it off to the manufacturers in Switzerland for repair.

It came back with an assurance it had been completely overhauled and was in perfect working order. Nevertheless, it continued to falter. With irritation, I sent it back a second time. The manufacturers returned it with a stiff little note saying their experts could find no fault and enclosed a catalogue of their new range.

A colleague suggested trying it on the other arm, with some dubious explanation about body electricity and magnetic fields. I put the watch on my right arm, and to my surprise, it worked. The half-scientific explanation troubled me slightly, but I was content that my treasured watch was now functional and I didn't give it another thought for the next year. It was then that I discovered there was nothing wrong with my self-winding watch and no mysterious electrical current was affecting it.

Instead, I discovered there was something wrong with my arm. It was when I was getting out of bed late on a Saturday morning in October 1970 that I noticed that my left arm was in continuous spasm. Soon a tremor replaced the spasm and I panicked. I did a rough test on myself; I stretched both arms in front of me parallel to the floor, to see whether there still was a tremor or whether it had been a momentary happening. The tremor continued. My first thought was of a cerebellar tumour. I phoned our GP. He invited me to come and see him that afternoon at his home instead of waiting until after the weekend to visit him at his surgery.

I told my wife, Lili, that I would have to be late for our four-year-old son's birthday party. My family knew that their father made little of aches and pains. 'We will watch it' was my stoic reaction to such things, and 'it will be all right in the morning', was my usual notorious response, in keeping with the course of masterly inactivity ingrained in me by an old-fashioned consultant at my medical school. Lili suspected, therefore, that something might be seriously wrong, but went on with her preparations for the children's party.

On my way to the Highgate home of our GP, I drove past Kenwood Park, one of the loveliest in North London, and the scene of many Sunday family outings, winter and summer. Now the chestnut trees were turning bright yellow, splashing their polished conkers on the pavement. I reflected that my life would be a short one and I was sad.

Michael Modell listened sympathetically and then went through the abbreviated neurological examination: tapping my reflexes, making me stretch my arms parallel to the ground and observing it all with a keen eye. He finished up looking with an opthalmoscope into my eyes and assured me that there were no signs of raised intracranial pressure, which would have shown a space-occupying lesion. He said he felt certain it was early Parkinson's disease. Strangely, this had not crossed my mind. He then comforted me with one advantage of PD; less likelihood of cardiac disease according to statistics. My later experience was to cast doubt on this.

Michael had been our family doctor from the time we returned to England from the United States, and I trusted his judgment and his reassuring words. Nevertheless, he insisted that I had the diagnosis confirmed and that the investigations for an essential base line should be made by a consultant neurologist at the London Hospital.

I was so relieved at not having a terminal brain tumour that anything less was welcome, especially as, in time and space, the end point seemed so far removed for the newly diagnosed sufferer. For me, Parkinson's disease recalled the shuffling, drooling and speech-affected old men and women in the outpatients' departments at hospitals where I had worked. I couldn't imagine myself in this role. From the viewpoint of a healthy thirty-nine year-old there remained a vast distance to cover.

I drove back through the golden autumn day, to our house where the children were popping balloons and passing the parcel. I joined in the game, not fully aware that I was about to embark on a more significant and preoccupying life game.

That night in bed, I suddenly understood why my watch

hadn't worked; its mechanism depended upon rhythmic swinging of the arm to wind itself. Not only was something wrong with my arm – I remembered the cramps I had experienced in my back while driving along the flat, monotonous Jutland roads, during our summer holiday on a Danish farm. The mosaic was beginning to fall into place.

But not quite. The overriding thought in my mind was why me, and why at this time? To find an answer to this riddle I was to dedicate all my attention and interest in the twenty years to come.

Next morning, I went back to my job at the Queen Elizabeth Hospital, East London, where I had just been appointed to the prestigious post of Consultant Child Psychiatrist. The requirements of the routine in a busy East End children's hospital forced the weekend's events out of my mind. A week later, I went for my appointment with Dr Henson who confirmed the diagnosis. I was relieved that he said it was minimal and that I was to go away and forget about it.

In the period of waiting, after the diagnosis was made and before I started medication, there were indications that the Parkinsonian process was developing. I recall a meeting with forty GPs from the area around Barnet Hospital where I was consulting. I was to make a clinical presentation, together with the social worker on the case, of the diagnostic and therapeutic work done with the family of a disturbed child. I had some notes for the presentation but rather grandly thought I would extemporize. I never fully considered how I would begin.

I stood up and had a complete mental block for about a minute, unable to think or to talk. I excused myself and went out of the room while the social worker took over. I caught my breath, and after five minutes rejoined the social worker. We completed the presentation together.

I remember sharing with him the fact that I had recently

been diagnosed as having Parkinson's disease. I felt that there was some secret about my body, which was confused with other secrets, and that the recent humiliation which I had experienced drove me to release the pressure. It was clear I was sitting on a keg of dynamite holding back the secret, together with a long line of secrets from the past – my mother's death, my father's remarriage and my own first marriage figured prominently in this list.

I made sure after this event that I was always fully prepared for future presentations.

The months passed and it slowly sank in that at thirty-nine, at the emerging peak of my professional career, with a third baby about to be born, I did indeed have Parkinson's disease, and that sooner or later it was going to interfere with my life's activities. I now set out on my single-minded pursuit to find out everything there was to know about the illness. The fact that no one had ever been known to be cured of it was a spur to my manic, omnipotent thinking. I even contemplated winning the Nobel prize for my research.

I began by renewing my knowledge of neurology as never before, studying in depth areas which, until now, I had merely been examined on. I scrutinized medical literature and wrote away for many reprints dealing with PD. Access to colleagues willing to discuss their research set me on my way to trying things out on myself. I searched for references to PD in pharmacological and medical journals. Friends from all over the world, knowing of my interest, scanned the lay press and started up a clipping service. I involved drug companies who were happy and willing on finding an educated guinea pig.

Most significantly of all, my training as a psychiatrist and psychoanalyst directed my wish to explore the interaction of the organic and the psychologically determined behaviour, present and past. In my psychoanalytic work I was deeply involved with the interface of body and mind, and in the future would have an opportunity to put to the test the theory long dawning on me, of the psychosomatic nature of my illness.

Just as James Parkinson had looked forward to understanding the development of the symptoms of the illness, Freud would encourage one to look back into the area of early development to evaluate a contribution from childhood.

CHAPTER 2

Parkinson's Disease

James Parkinson, who first diagnosed and gave Parkinson's disease its name, wrote in his preface to *The Shaking Palsy* in 1817 that, 'the disease is of long duration: To connect, therefore, the symptoms which occur in its later stages with those which mark its commencement, requires a continuance of observation of the same case, or at least a correct history of its symptoms, even for several years'.

My intention in writing this book is to record the first twenty years of a protracted course of Parkinson's disease.

Idiopathic Parkinson's disease (PD of unknown origin) is a chronic degenerative disorder affecting at least one in a thousand of the population, ten per cent having the onset before the age of forty. Men and women are equally affected, and no nationality or ethnic group is spared.

The site of the disorder is mainly in the basal ganglia of the brain where, for reasons still unclear, dopaminergic nigral cells die in the substantia nigra and fail to secrete the neurotransmitter, dopamine, which transmits signals to other brain cells and instructs them to initiate movement. Depletion of dopamine in the corpus striatum, the section of the brain which is responsible for the motor effects of the disease, follows. By the time it comes to medical attention, eighty per cent of the total number of these cells will no longer be secreting dopamine.

Patients with PD suffer a gradual loss of motor functions, with slowness of movement leading to akinesia, rigidity, tremor, gait disturbance and loss of postural reflexes affecting balance. In time, secondary effects emerge, with speech losing volume and handwriting shrinking in size. Eventually, symptoms occur affecting coordination and flow of movement between the two sides of the body. The simplest of tasks, such as tying a shoe lace or turning over in bed, become insuperable.

The advent in 1967 of the drug, L-dopa, has altered the natural history of the illness, extending life-expectation close to the norm. But the effect of the illness on quality of life remains considerable. L-dopa is a precursor of the neurotransmitter, dopamine, whose metabolism and transfer is disturbed in the Parkinsonian brain. Since dopamine itself cannot cross the blood-brain barrier in treatment, L-dopa is given to replenish the deficiency of the brain's own residual production, which diminishes in the process of the disease.

Since the early days of treatment with this pill, new drugs based on new principles have evolved. Dopamine agonists, which directly stimulate the brain's dopamine receptors, have been developed and put to trial and use. The specialist neurologist is constantly having to keep ahead of his patient's needs, but until it is fully understood why the cells degenerate, PD is likely to remain a puzzle. Understanding the cause of degeneration will benefit newly diagnosed patients more than old stagers like myself. Meanwhile, I think it important for patients to record the events of their illness, so as to make their personal map of the territory available to those who follow. There are various reasons for this, of which caution is one, but mainly it is to avoid participating in hare-brained schemes in pursuit of a cure.

This work began as an essay that was intended to find the relationship, if any, between illness and personality. With the orientation of my training as a psychoanalyst, I looked at my origins and early childhood experience and found in it significant elements of depression and loss. The response of people to my publication of a personal study lent strong support to this thesis, and many of the letters I received stated that in their Parkinson's disease, too, loss of someone close had been implicated. It also alerted me to the paucity of published material written by patients with PD.

In seeking to chronicle my past, it is my intention to stimulate Parkinsonian readers to explore their own history and to enable them to find its relevance, if any, to the early symptoms of the disease. While not altering its course, this exploration will make the condition more liveable with, because understood. It will describe experiences which would have been avoided had wise counsel been available to the writer. Such counselling would, first and foremost, recognize and handle depression in its various forms in PD, as well as its playing partners, the precarious and insubstantial flights into health.

While reviewing the literature on PD and personality, I discovered that many psychiatrists found a common core of personality among PD sufferers, much of it ante-dating the onset of the illness by as much as twenty-five years and longer. This book will illustrate the co-existence of the factor of early loss and the depression that arises as a consequence of it, often compounded across three generations.

The knowledge of where one stands in relation to an illness makes a mystery tolerable rather than fearful. It also helps in orienting oneself with the stage one has reached at any particular time.

I offer this work, then, as coming from special vantage points; that of psychoanalysis, with a look at emotional development from infancy to adulthood; and of psychiatry, with the recognition of states of mind, mood, continuity and causation. Both of these views contribute to an understanding of the doctor-patient relationship about which I have critical comments to make throughout the book. It is rare to find oneself in such a privileged position, and I hope I may do justice to that position.

CHAPTER 3

Growing Up in South Africa

Yeoville, where I was born, is a suburb of Johannesburg, South Africa, the city that grew up at the centre of the ridge of gold-containing ore discovered in 1886. It was developed by speculators after World War I and named after a city councillor, Yeo, with a French ending added. In the 1930s, it was a charmless, would-be garden suburb, a fifteen-minute tram ride away from the city centre. It was laid out in a grid and was conspicuous for the dreariness of its architecture. The bungalows, too big for the plots they were built on, had garages attached to the outhouses for the servants. They were memorials to middle-class pretentions.

So were the street names, resonant of the great names of English aristocratic families: Fortescue, Raleigh, Bedford, Cavendish, Dunbar and Grafton, with a couple of undistinguished Dutch names thrown in.

These street names, in white on blue enamel, were the first letters that I saw when I graduated to a push chair from an oversprung, giant-wheeled landau, inherited from my brother and sister, from which I could see only the sky above. Unlike the nannies of other Yeoville families, mine was white and of Boer origin. Gertie was a nubile eighteen year-old when she joined our family a few months before my birth; she stayed with us for eight years.

I discovered, years later, that my mother's pregnancy had been beset by problems. Her father had died in the early stages, probably leaving her depressed and sad. Then, as the result of an accident six months into pregnancy, she was further shocked and dispirited. My father, a mechanically naive man, had overturned our hearse-like sedan on an outing to the country. Everyone survived, but when I was born my mother was debilitated and had great difficulty in feeding me.

My mother's own mother had died in Russia giving birth to her; and her father, an erudite and scholarly man, but no provider as a husband, remarried a young woman with regal bearing who took over the running of his family. Together, they added another two babies. His three eldest daughters went to America to join relatives there, while my grandfather took the rest of his brood to South Africa in an endeavour to make a living. His work included running a bakery and managing a cinema which he owned, called 'The Good Hope'. Inevitably things went wrong when he was at the helm and they struggled.

My father, who had come out to South Africa at the tender age of sixteen, was a great admirer of the learned improviser, and married his daughter. She was the central figure in the family and helped support them with her work in a shipping insurance office.

My mother's stepmother whom I knew as 'Bobby', was an imposing, handsome woman who always kept me well supplied with jelly babies. Her brother, Isaac, a furrier from Paris who visited in 1936 with his radium-scarred and grafted face and his tales of the Folies Bergère provided an exotic connection with Europe. A seasoned bachelor, his skin defect, like that of the *Phantom of the Opera*, greatly affected his life. He returned to Johannesburg to settle there permanently after the outbreak of war. I recall the grey spats and the fact that, like a true Frenchman, he didn't bathe but daubed himself with great bottles of Cologne water. The two largest stamps in my collection came from letters that he had sent, and depicted a heavily moustached Maréchal Joffre.

Our fishmonger was named Joffe, a most unmilitary Jew, who I imagined was related to the man on the stamp. The latter would chop the Friday evening fish on a sawn-up tree trunk, the heads would fall into a bucket from which the eyes stared out, ready for a cat's meal. The shop was one of two dozen in the High Street, through which the tram cars clanged on their way to and from the city. I would go there with my nurse, Gertie, and occasionally with my mother.

For the next ten years following his accident in the car, my father didn't trust himself to drive. We relied on Checker and Yellow cabs which were the familiar mode of transport for Sunday outings. There was also an occasional ride in an open sports car driven by a swashbuckling uncle who resembled Erroll Flynn. Better still, there were rides in the dicky seat. I would step up to this inverted boot, where the wind swept through my hair on the open road, and if I managed to put the rumble out of my mind, I could commune with the gods and the spirits of the wind.

Every Saturday afternoon I was packed off with Gertie to

the Yeoville cinema. For the price of a sixpenny ticket, and one and a penny for Gertie, I was given access to this elderly picture palace where one could dream the impossible while identifying with the screen offering for the afternoon. This then was the South African bioscope, which took its name from one of the companies that made the early silent movies and gave its name to cinemas throughout the country.

My timidity was protected by Gertie's presence, about which I had mixed feelings – I would have preferred holding my own against some of the tough kids who, unaccompanied by nannies, sat with their big brothers. Mine was seven years older than me and clearly thought himself in another league when it came to going to the bioscope.

I recall vividly some of the movie stars I saw, including Buck Jones, Tom Mix, Fred Astaire and Ginger Rogers. A film I specially liked was *The Great Waltz* about Johann Strauss, and this brought me my first awareness of Vienna which was to become a recurring theme in my life. Jeanette McDonald, abandoned by Allan Jones singing *The Donkey Serenade*, was Gertie's favourite and our house was filled with her bellowing imitation of it.

My mother played the piano with strong rhythm, and while she was playing, I danced. *The Waves of the Danube* and an aria from *Rigoletto* were her specialities.

In Muizenberg, where we spent our annual summer holidays in January, I relished playing in the cool bleached sand with my bucket and spade. One summer, when I was recovering from a serious attack of pneumonia, I was forced to wear my imported Jaeger vest, buttoned right up to the throat, the minute I emerged from the lovely cool water. My body seemed to be the centre of concern for the adults as, the year before, I had had my tonsils removed with the complication of repeated haemorrhages. My body image was a distinctly weedy one but in my mind it was transformed by my fantasies of great strength and power.

Somehow, the direct experience of pleasure was always inhibited by the grown-ups' nagging. My older brother and sister belonged in another world, where everything seemed to me to be permitted. They were not compelled to go for a nap in the early afternoon, nor, in the evening when everything promised to be at its liveliest, were they required to leave abruptly for bed. Visitors arriving for a card party on a Saturday night would sometimes sneak into my bedroom and give me a hug and some of my favourite Aero chocolate. I recall the present of a rough-hewn tennis racquet, lacking in gloss and strung with ordinary string, but a remarkably treasured possession to sleep with alongside my teddy bear.

Thursday was nurse Gertie's afternoon off. It was my time alone with my mother and, after our shopping was completed, we visited friends or relatives. Instead of sitting in the kitchen or the back porch with other guardians of the young and their charges, I was allowed to have my tea in the front lounge.

My mother died in 1938, in the month that Hitler's tanks rolled into Vienna. My sister, three years older than myself, now accompanied me to the shops instead of my mother.

That bare statement overlies the most shattering and significant event in my life. My mother's death came immediately after an operation for gall stones, neglected for years because of her fear of 'the knife'. By the time she was operated on, her liver was a mass of abscesses and failed completely a few days later.

No one had thought to keep me informed about the seriousness of my mother's situation. Nor was I taken to see her after the operation. I was left at the age of six-plus mystified by what had happened. Children then were not expected to be aware of such matters.

This mystification was compounded by the daily prayers said in our home, over a week-long period after her death, by the rest of the family and friends in the Jewish community. Pictures were removed and mirrors covered. The mourners, other than myself, sat in elected discomfort on upturned mineral water crates. I saw it all as a game, and just as I did with the people who used to come visiting in the past, I would badger the tall men to lift me high onto their shoulders. In this way, I could touch the ceiling and could continue to behave as before, only this time having more reason to reach for the sky. I assumed my mother's spirit was floating about up there. At night, crying myself to sleep, I thought of a body rotting in a coffin in the ground. Would some sort of *sutie* be expected of me? Why had I been excluded from the funeral? Can one really be too young at six to be sure that any deadly spirits are sealed off and reparative feelings initiated? 'The sorrow that does not out in tears makes other organs weep'. These words attributed to Henry Maudsley, the great nineteenth-century psychiatrist, come to mind now, leaving me with no doubt that through long consolidated pathways of subsequent experience, my Parkinson's disease represents that weeping function.

I coped with the cold and the absence of love at seven by dividing my bed into two halves, sleeping in the warm cosy half and avoiding the cold, rejected split-off other half. The technique of distancing myself from real feelings, combined with the avoidance of pain, left me in cloud-cuckoo-land.

Significantly, my mother's death occurred three weeks before my seventh birthday in May 1938, and spoilt subsequent birthdays forever for me.

At the same time, the news bulletins on the wireless were strident with the events of the war in Europe. It was the beginning of a siege that ended, for most, in 1945, but for me there was an ambiguity; the happy ending I would have wanted was not to be found. And the inner war continued.

Two weeks after her death I returned to school and was bullied because of my absence. There was a smallpox epidemic and pupils who had been vaccinated against it wore red armbands. I wore a black armband, as a sign of mourning, but this failed to deter a bully called Gallow from sinking his fist into my arm, raw from its vaccinations. I never forgave him and was glad when his family moved away and he left the school the following year.

My father remarried two years later, heeding my grand-mother's advice that 'the children need a mother'. I was pleased to again have a mother like all the other boys and we agreed that I call her aunt Sarah. I quite liked her and looked forward to enjoying life again. I was relieved when she found that she couldn't bear Gertie, who was soon dismissed; I secretly hoped that this would free me from being treated like a baby.

Sarah was a second generation South African, more assimilated than my father but still familiar with the Sabbath ritual and the Jewish holiday celebrations. She'd been a piano teacher before she married my father and it was important to me that she could play the sheet music that had been assembled in our house over the years.

This activity was one further continuity of the old order which I relished. She asked my brother, sister and myself what we thought about her having children. None of us were thrilled with the idea. She was forty when she married and we needn't have worried. She had to wait till the birth of my sister's children to practice her infant-mothering skills. In the meantime, I continued in the privileged role as 'her baby'.

She had a delightful sense of humour and told a story well. She also taught me how to play contract bridge and was pleased when I won a newspaper competition. Two years after she came to our house, a powder-blue Dodge car was bought. She had lessons and passed her driving test. Later my father, too, returned to driving. It was she, however, who took the wheel when the family went down to East London, a two-day trip of about 800 miles through some mountainous terrain, a journey requiring courage and skill and I admired her for it.

When she first arrived, I was eight-and-a-half and she continued the practice of bathing me once a week. I found this very exciting and would come to the bathroom with a proud member. Sarah's Victorian background dictated her response to this intimate display and she would wash my back and then tell me to wash between the legs, as if to confirm that there was something eminently male that was being overlooked.

In my behaviour with friends and family, I was rigid and unyielding, sporting a front that was precociously aimed at trying to scale a half generation in order to be included among my older brother's and sister's circle of friends. Quarrels with my classmates were drawn out and I lacked the ability to recover from being hurt. All my defences foundered when I was put to any test, revealing real immaturity and a learning block. My barmitzvah found me nervously anticipating that portion of the law I was required to sing and the large family party I had to attend after the synagogue service. There was also another party on the following day. I developed a temperature of 102° and an earache which quickly disappeared within the half hour. I did what was expected of me and even made a short speech.

Socially, as I moved into the teenage years, life was awkward, dominated by irrational forces that I couldn't control. I recall a mixed party given by my favourite girl cousin when I was sixteen. I wore my school blazer and an imported Tootal tie of pre-war manufacture, which in my eyes made it very desirable and important. Everyone else at the party was relaxed in flannels and sports shirts. I was right out of my generation. I felt bashful, waited in a side room, and wouldn't go into the party until near the end, by which time most of the other guests had left.

In creative matters, I was unable to let fly and come up with imaginative work. Instead, I compromised and produced self-conscious and wooden patterns. For example, when our art teacher gave us each a ceramic tile to decorate, I could think of nothing better to paint than my initials, neatly and accurately measured with a ruler. In this concrete-thinking way I suppressed any unpredictable or sensual elements in myself.

One Monday in 1948 when I was seventeen, our class was to be tested on the subject of the 1815 Congress of Vienna. I felt sympathy for Napoleon, exiled to St Helena, and Metternich also caught my imagination as the grand designer of the congress. The exam was to be followed by an inter-school debate in which I was to present the motion 'Human Nature Never Changes'. The combination of pressures were too much for me and I had an attack of the jitters before writing the essay. It took me ten minutes to calm myself and get over it and it sensitized me to exams: I spent the next sixteen years one way or another sitting exams, presumably in part, to counter the phobia of being tested.

When it came to choosing my career, the same lack of imagination determined my choice. I would have liked to follow in the footsteps of my brother and study medicine. But coping with unconsciousness and death was too threatening at this crucial time of adolescence. Disregarding my friends' opinions that dentistry was boring, I chose to become a dentist. In South Africa, dentists are given the title doctor; they also enjoy fixed hours, are not called out at night and make a good living.

I spent five years at Witwatersrand University in the

dental faculty. While the rest of the university, and the medical school in particular, prided itself on its liberal policies, with blacks among its students, the dental department was run more like a penal colony than an academic institution. The discipline was fierce and the full-time supervisors devastating in their application of it. Everything we did was noted in our record book which had a special section for adverse comments. It was little wonder that there were two suicides among the students in my year.

In the third year, when we began to do extractions, I was confronted with a heavily built African who pointed to an enormous but decayed molar tooth in his upper jaw. I injected the area and, after a while, laid the forceps onto the tooth, pushing them up between the gum and the bone in a solid grip. Then I began to swing at the end of the forceps, to no avail. I called the supervisor who had a gammy leg and propelled himself with the aid of a crutch; as a consequence the muscle in his right arm was massive. He did everything I had done with ten times the amount of force. Suddenly, there was a loud crack. We looked down to see the forceps had broken, while the tooth defiantly remained in place. The patient, who by then had had enough, jumped out of the chair saying in Zulu: *mininga chiesa* (very hot). The supervisor, not to be trifled with, pushed him back into the chair saying, 'If you don't behave, I'll make you pay for the forceps!' I proceeded to extract the tooth with a heavier pair of forceps. It was not perhaps the most sympathetic environment in which to learn about a caring profession.

In my final year, in the orthodontic exam, I experienced my second attack of jitters. I couldn't hold together two wires that required soldering. Again much effort at relaxation was needed to overcome this problem and continue with the exam.

CHAPTER 4

Growing Up Again in London

I hurried overseas in 1954, soon after qualifying, avoiding the graduation ceremony, with its symbolic maturation, and escaping the confinement and insularity of the South African scene. I left never dreaming I was leaving permanently, nor that when I returned on my last visit, twenty-five years later, it would be to talk as an expert on Parkinson's disease.

I had not been involved politically, but no one could avoid being aware of the almost daily incidents in which blacks were subjected to degradation, humiliation and rough handling. They tolerated this with remarkable courage –

even managing a sense of humour. But it was one law for the blacks and one for the whites well before apartheid became the official law after 1948. The paradox was that the whites, who prided themselves on being Europeans, had little of the culture of true Europeans.

There were many jobs available for dentists in the British NHS, which had come into operation five years earlier. I sailed from Cape Town on the *ss Winchester Castle*, seen off by my father and stepmother, who were vacationing there, and by my girlfriend who lived there. She and I had met a couple of years earlier when I was taking a holiday break in the middle of my dental course. When I qualified, we met again and spent time together. We were just beginning to know one another when I left for England. We corresponded during the first three years of my stay.

The first job I took was as an assistant to a dentist in North London. I hated the work, the confinement of the site, as well as the premises. Being thrown on my own standards, after the experience of a jail-like dental hospital, left me floundering and unhappy. Within six months of arriving, I was seeing my first psychotherapist, and talking about changing professions to medicine. As a compromise I did post-graduate dentistry and orthodontics and still talked about enrolling in medical school.

I moved from a depressing lodging with my brother and his wife in Willesden Green to London House, a comfortable, well-appointed residence for Commonwealth students in the centre of Bloomsbury. While there I completed my dental fellowship, studies and exams.

The three years' correspondence with my girlfriend had brought us close to an understanding when, in the flush of exuberance after passing the Fellowship of Dental Surgery finals, I wrote to her revealing that I had taken the decision to study medicine with a view to becoming a psychiatrist. She replied, praising the first part of the decision, but adding a note of caution about the psychiatry, saying that she felt that it was still in its early days and that like early workers in the field of X-rays, there was a strong possibility of getting one's fingers burnt. With the advantage of thirty-four years of hindsight, I would say that it was good advice.

However, at the time, I was in a turmoil and in a fragile state of mind. I took her advice as a slap in the face and a failure to really understand me. My turmoil was caused by the sudden death of my psychotherapist while I was on holiday the previous autumn, which left me in a state of deep dependency, not fully comprehended by his successor.

That evening, flushed with success, I bumped into a friend, a South African poet, in a favourite restaurant of ours, the 'Old Vienna'. The paprika chicken, the Wiener schnitzel and fried chicken liver with onions reminded everyone of home. When he said he was going to the Lyceum dance hall, I agreed to accompany him. This was my first visit to such a place; I was more familiar with the Saturday night college hops. I was primed to do something stupid that evening; I wasn't to know that there was a woman out there in the dance hall who was equally primed and even more so. Lydia was engaged to be married to an American in a month's time and, with one failed marriage behind her, felt very uncertain of herself. We met and married in record time, before the letter from my girlfriend arrived in which she apologised for her criticism of my choice of career.

The turnabout, from a promising three-year relationship to a precipitous marriage in three weeks, had something to do with a wish to hurt everyone around me, just as I had been left out and hurt. It certainly had nothing to do with love.

We were married at the Paddington registry office on a Saturday in September. On Sunday morning I woke up to the realization that I had made a ghastly mistake in thinking that I could mature by such an action. I had agreed to marry her because I couldn't bear to let her go, and she had insisted that if I didn't marry her by special licence, she would marry her fiancé as planned. For three months I lived with her in a small rented flat, discovering that she had told me less than the truth, and by the New Year I had set in motion steps for our divorce.

I was left licking my wounds in an embarrassed withdrawal from social life for another two years, waiting for my divorce. By then I had decided that instead of returning to my old university to switch to medicine, I would stay in London, and enrolled at the West London Hospital in Hammersmith. The compulsion to become a psychiatrist was now irresistible and took on the character of a mission.

I was grateful that I had studied the full anatomy, physiology and pathology courses as part of my dental training in Johannesburg; this was recognized by the examining board and I was only required to do three clinical years to qualify.

I spent the three years as a student helping to earn my living by working part-time as a dentist up the road in Hammersmith. A number of fellow medical students came to me as dental patients. Doing dentistry as a means to an end, not permanently, even made it enjoyable. My fellow medical students were mainly mature students like myself, and included a Norwegian ship's captain, an Australian air line pilot, a BBC programmer and a host of people who had crashed out at some stage in their original hospital placements. Like me, they were 'rescued' by the dean, Maurice Shaw, and a team of consultants, who gave us all a second chance. The atmosphere was friendly and the place full of bar-room characters. One could always get a game of bridge at short notice. The medical school numbers among its distinguished alumni a former MP, who is at present a leading medical journalist, two senior medical politicians and many successful medical practitioners.

The school merged with Charing Cross, when that hospital moved to Fulham, and the original school ceased to exist. Now the alumni and former consultants, a shrinking crowd, meet once a year, while the building has been given over to an obstetric unit and may soon be closing as a consequence of cuts.

On passing my final exams, I got my first job in general medicine, neurology and psychiatry. My next job was at New End Hospital in the heart of Hampstead, an upgraded workhouse where I did surgery and gynaecology. Among its departments, it had an internationally famous thyroid unit. With the neighbourhood's population of creative and often disturbed people, there was a steady flow of overdosed patients requiring resuscitation. One night I had to go to the mortuary to identify and confirm the death of a man whose head was lying next to his feet. He had jumped in front of the tube train at the local station. I recall one Friday afternoon and evening in theatre when a seven-year-old boy was admitted; he had fallen across a broken glass flower cloche in his garden, cutting a femoral artery in his groin. Although he was transfused with thirteen pints of blood, he couldn't be saved. Set against these hair-raising experiences, there was the satisfaction of assisting at routine abdominal surgery and performing hernia operations and appendectomies under supervision.

After finishing at New End, while contemplating a trip to America, I spent some months doing locum work and night calls, seeing, incidentally, parts of London I had not previously known. It was a relaxed period in my life which I needed, having driven myself relentlessly. Theatres and concerts were my choice for relaxation and enjoyment.

I also worked again as a dental locum while awaiting replies from job applications in psychiatry in the United

States. It was in the dentist's office where I was filling in a session one morning, that the girl who became my wife walked into the surgery for an emergency appointment for a broken tooth. Her name was Lili Loebl and she was over from the United States visiting her mother in northern England. She had an engaging personality and a charming smile. I asked her about her work at the United Nations where she was a correspondent for *Newsweek* magazine. I remember feeling moved by the murder that autumn of Dag Hammarskjold, the Secretary General, when his plane was shot down over Africa. She left me her card when I said I was planning to visit the United States. I now had an additional reason for looking forward to my journey.

I had no fixed appointment waiting for me when I arrived in New York, but had arranged interviews and had passed the ECFMG (Educational Certificate for Foreign Medical Graduates), with which one would be allowed to practise as a doctor in American hospitals.

I visited Hillside Hospital on Long Island, and was most impressed by their dynamic approach and in-service training. I was there for a year which was spent instructively in the refined ambiance of a therapeutic community supervised by experienced psychoanalysts in the treatment of patients; and there I learnt in depth about mental illness. My spare time was spent in the company of Lili. This was a period of great political activity centred around the United Nations and I joined her in much of the social life which accompanied her pursuit of stories.

For my second year in the United States, I moved to Boston where I did a further year of residency (registrarship) in the outpatients' department of the busy City Hospital. Here, as well as seeing the seamy, alcoholic and violent side of the New World, I experienced the warmth and welcome of the medical fraternity at the Harvard service to which I was attached.

It was in the hospital's former mortuary, reclaimed by a Greek fellow psychiatric registrar as his preferred lodging, that we all watched the events following the assassination of John Kennedy on TV. Nibbling on feta cheese, olives and sweetmeats, provided by our host, we saw with horror the transfer of Lee Harvey Oswald from his cell and the live killing of Kennedy's 'assassin'.

One weekend, I was returning from a skiing trip in Vermont with some friends, when we ran over an elk crossing the highway in Connecticut. Repairs to the radiator were necessary, and in a small village nearby we found a garage. Next to it, in a car dealer's lot, I noticed a black Renault for sale at one hundred dollars, which was as much as I could afford. I inquired about it and was told by a mechanic that the owner was a Seventh Day Adventist and would not do any business until six o'clock after the Sabbath had ended. I waved my friends on and paced in the freezing cold for three hours. At six o'clock sharp an elegantly suited gentleman appeared and the transaction took place. It was the first car I ever owned. I drove off and soon discovered that the car had no brakes and that I was forced, for my survival, to rely on the hand brake. It was a terrifying trip back to New York and presumably the zealot put in a special prayer of thanks to his Lord for having delivered up such a timely sucker.

I also discovered some members of my scattered tribe. The name Todes is not very common, so I was surprised when I arrived in Boston to discover a Todes, initials S.J. We met for a beer in a bar off Harvard Square. He was a philosophy professor at MIT and shared my delight at this meeting. He mentioned that his father, who was director of Hebrew education in Rochester, NY, would be visiting New York for the weekend before Christmas and we arranged to meet under the clock at Grand Central Station. Inside the Biltmore Hotel, with the snow thick outside, I became acquainted with this most impressive man. In his late sixties, David Todes was lean and sinewy and looked at one with alert piercing eyes. I spent a riveting afternoon in his company while he recounted the family history and his own adventures with T.E. Lawrence in Arabia.

In early 1964, together with my wife-to-be, I flew on a brief trip to London where I was accepted for psychoanalytic studies. The four- to five-year training course was to start in September.

My dental experience had one final positive fallout: at Tufts University I was given permission to use gold-casting apparatus to fashion the wedding ring.

We were married on Long Island at the home of a former colleague of Lili. It was a beautiful day, with the ceremony held in the garden under a *chupah*, woven in cornflowers and marguerites by a Hindu friend familiar with the custom. A band played and we danced and had a wonderful send off for our honeymoon on the *ss France* bound for England.

I had arrived in America with one suitcase, and was returning with a Harvard chair wrapped up in a Persian rug, the painting of a magic animal by a Catalan friend, ten pieces of luggage and a wife. These all had to be carried up to the attic apartment in Hampstead, which we had rented through an advertisement in the *New Statesman*, and competed for space with a huge brass bed and a collection of stuffed animals belonging to Beryl Bainbridge, our landlady *in absentia*. She was on holiday in Greece, and on her return became one of our first friends in England.

I found a job as a psychiatrist in the British equivalent of a therapeutic community at Halliwick Hospital and began my psychoanalytic training. As soon as there was a vacancy, I went to work in the children's department at the Tavistock Clinic where John Bowlby was based. His stress on the significance of the child's attachment to the mother was revolutionizing the care of children in hospitals and institutions, as well as making a language for use in everyday psychotherapeutic work. His theory touched me profoundly because of my own experience of losing my mother, and it influenced the quality and pattern of parenting of my children.

Towards the end of my psychoanalytic training, I was offered a post at the Hampstead Child Therapy Clinic doing diagnostic work and taking part in a number of research projects. This was a most stimulating environment. There was close contact with American psychoanalysts who valued the set-up more than the local fraternity.

Anna Freud presided over the clinic and was its inspirational source. She was having an Indian summer of productivity, and attending her seminars and workshops and preparing her developmental diagnostic profiles was a unique learning experience. She was the coordinating brain behind each and every sentence that came out of the clinic. She was conversant with the day-to-day progress of each of the sixty patients who were in five times a week treatment with staff and students; moreover, she had them cross-referenced in her mind better than any computer and certainly better than any of us.

The plenary clinic meetings she chaired and the public lectures she gave, saw her wooing her audience in her clear high-pitched voice with its precise vocabulary and faintest trace of Viennese accent. She never referred to notes. In her mid-seventies when I joined the clinic, her bent-over figure with the silver hair and the dark ankle-length skirts which she made herself, was a familiar sight crossing over Maresfield Gardens to her home (now the Freud Museum, since her death in 1982).

She had changed nothing there since Freud died in 1939 and here in his study where she held teaching seminars, she received her guests, psychoanalysts, academics and politicians. For a student in psychoanalysis it was a unique setting. I was there until 1977 by which time my own ideas on a whole-patient approach conflicted with Miss Freud's concept. She saw herself as standing guard over the inheritance of psychoanalysis to which she had dedicated her life and made a unique contribution. In the end she was limited, as lesser and greater mortals, by the times in which she had been brought up.

CHAPTER 5

Death in Vienna

In April 1971, my family was completed with the birth of a daughter, Ariane. We were living in a huge rented flat high up in Hampstead. It had communal gardens and on a clear day you could see as far as the Chiltern hills. Soon after, my father who had been widowed again two years earlier, was well enough to make his first trip outside of South Africa since he had emigrated from Lithuania at the age of sixteen.

He was now in his early eighties and was accompanied by my brother for a three-week stay. We had good and precious moments together, making me regret that I had had such poor contact with him over the years. He was a man of great integrity and sense of justice. He was especially pleased to help with baby sitting when the chaos in the expanded household required his help, and proudly rocked his granddaughter to sleep with an old Yiddish lullaby 'Rosinkes and Mandelen' (Raisins and Almonds). But the peak of his pleasure was a trip to 'Scotland', which had been his dream for many years.

In the event, we stretched the Scottish border more accessibly south, close to Newcastle and substituted the Cheviot foothills for the lowlands of Scotland. We stayed with my mother-in-law who was a flirtatious and stylish hostess and enabled his dream to come true. He died two years later without ever knowing of my illness.

My training analysis had ended not long after qualifying as a psychoanalyst in 1968. With the onset of PD in 1971, I returned to my analyst, Dr Lothair Rubinstein, thinking that he would have some understanding of the significance of the condition from his long experience with me. Surprisingly, he was more concerned with its organic aspect, while I pretended to myself that there were not any physical or structural defects. As in hysteria, I felt that conflict within myself was responsible for producing this left-handed tremor which, so far, was the only noticeable symptom. He recommended I see another neurologist, Dr Simon Behrman, for confirmation. He nearly fell off his chair when I recited to him my daily timetable of commitments, and pointed out that I had driven myself from exam to exam, with dentistry moving into dental fellowship and orthodontics to medicine and psychiatry. I had to agree with him, but I didn't see any alternative at this stage with a growing family.

A few months later, Rubinstein was dead, the possibilities of discussing things further with him no longer existed. But the event of his passing needs recounting.

Rubinstein and I attended the International Psychoanalytic Congress in Vienna that summer. It was a special one; the first such congress to welcome back Anna Freud to the country which had unceremoniously kicked out her and her illustrious father in 1938, after the Anschluss. Everyone was excited about the event. Dr Rubinstein, too, had left in 1938 and going back must have been tremendously stressful. An additional stress factor was a threatened secession of the Hampstead Clinic, under Miss Freud, from the British Psychoanalytic Society to become an autonomous institute.

An extraordinary meeting of the clinic staff was called in the gilded side room of the Hofburg Palace ballroom at lunchtime on the opening day of the congress, to discuss this schism and to test out support. Dr Rubinstein, who was in both camps, spoke in favour of maintaining links with the British society and soon after finishing talking, collapsed and gave a few stertorous gasps, as he rapidly lost consciousness. Two other medical colleagues and I rushed over to him and, without any conscious thought, I found myself giving mouth to mouth respiration to my analyst, while Clifford Yorke, clinic director, pummelled his chest and moved his arms to ventilate the lungs. The rest of the meeting withdrew to let us proceed with the attempted resuscitation, which was proving fruitless. An analyst who was also a GP came into the room and confirmed that he was dead.

I didn't seem to feel much anxiety then, nor did I at the cemetery two days later when he was cremated. This was a response to shock which, despite all my analysis, left me remote from the deep underlying feeling in the face of severe loss. There was a *déjà vu* about these gravelled paths crunching under foot between the alleys of trees. The cemetery had not changed in twenty-five years since the film of *The Third Man* was made there. I left my colleagues and walked back to the car with my thoughts about Dr Rubinstein and the tragedy for his family.

I found Vienna haunting. For me, there was the association of the earlier Congress of Vienna, and of course the link with the origins of psychoanalysis. Then there was the music, the Strauss waltzes that my mother had played on our upright Steinway in Yeoville, and to which I had danced as a child. Lehar's *Merry Widow* was my father's favourite operetta, and Mozart and Mahler of later acquaintance. I visited the Theatre an der Wien, where Beethoven had conducted his first performance of *Fidelio*. All this nostalgia was a balm to my shocked system.

Nevertheless, the rest of the congress was coloured by the death. The association of the clinic and the society was amicably resolved and I was glad when I returned to London and found my family back from their holiday in Northumberland. I had bought my sons a Subuteo football game that we could play on a table-top, and a self-regulating car, and a silver thimble for my daughter's charm bracelet.

CHAPTER 6

Drug Holiday and Hospitalization

My search for a cure began in the autumn of 1971, a year after the diagnosis was made. Motivated by a need to find a solution, to be there before the illness would slow me, I was driven by a wish to keep up with my contemporaries. My ambitions were now divided between my job as a child psychiatrist and psychoanalyst, and my attempt to make a contribution to the understanding of Parkinson's disease. I also wanted, no doubt, to obscure my role as a patient.

I began writing to anyone who was an authority on PD, reading the literature and instructing myself about the relatively new treatment with L-dopa. This drug had been in general use only in the past five years, and the field was wide open. Certainly the knowledge of its efficacy, which had completely changed the expectation of treatment, tempered my anxiety about my illness.

L-dopa was first used in 1967 but, at the time of my diagnosis, it was only available in research centres. One centre where it was being used was the Hammersmith Hospital, where Donald Calne was doing pioneering work on PD. I came across his monograph on Parkinson's disease while browsing in Lewis' medical bookshop in Bloomsbury and bought a copy. It contained some of the original work on L-dopa, and Calne postulated that early treatment with the substance might retard the progress of the disease.

I contacted Dr Calne directly, a habit which, as a fellow consultant, I was to repeat many times over the years. This, in effect, bypassed my GP and landed me in the guise of a guinea pig – a predicament that might otherwise have been avoided by full discussion with my doctor.

My symptoms were still of the slightest, but, with prevention in mind and the current theory that large quantities of the drug might indeed retard the progression of Parkinson's disease, I stuffed myself with L-dopa in as large and many doses as I could tolerate, just short of producing the unwanted side effects of nausea, dyskinesia (grimacing) and hypotension (fainting). It was a fine line and I didn't always achieve it.

One of these attacks was at a cocktail party given by the Group Analytic Society in the low-ceilinged suite of an apartment mansion block in Marylebone. I felt everyone going round and round, my wife looking anxiously at me and guiding me out into the hallway for fresh air where I collapsed totally. I woke to find my pulse being taken by a colleague who was also loosening my tie.

I continued to reel under the drug regime, but was aware of the main benefit; my left arm was swinging voluntarily.

Dr Calne mentioned that the side effects were responding to the addition of carbi-dopa, an enzyme inhibitor which enabled smaller doses of L-dopa to be effective centrally, without causing nausea or hypotension. The name of the combined pill was Sinemet, deriving from its anti-emetic effect. Sinemet was being tested by David Marsden who had just been appointed to the chair of neurology at the Maudsley and King's College Hospital, and Dr Calne arranged for me to see him. Marsden was dispensing some very helpful medication and included me in his trials of Sinemet. Once it was generally available, I returned to Dr Calne.

I felt well and had a good response to the medication in the morning, part of the afternoon and the evening. The side effects were minimal, and I was prepared to face the future with the knowledge that new drugs were bound to emerge to bridge the gap. I was generally in a slightly elated state due to the L-dopa and I quite enjoyed this, although there were some moments of depression just before the drug became effective, and by the evening I usually felt fatigued.

I started playing tennis again after a long interruption. Also, on visiting the studio of a potter, where I was taken by a colleague, I was given a ball of clay and threw it on the wheel; I was surprised to discover that I had some ability for pottery and was happy to be taken on as a pupil.

The habit of introspection and self-scrutiny, so much part of my training as a psychoanalyst, was fortified by the need to keep summary charts of my medication and response. The peak was the tendency to awake at 4 a.m. with very clear thinking. Some model of a biological clock seemed to be operating to account for a different response to the same drug at different times.

I was working at Queen Elizabeth Hospital and Hoxton Child Guidance Clinic as well as one and a half days a week at the Hampstead Child Therapy Clinic. Travelling to work in the East End four days a week, often through rush hours, began to leave me fatigued. A colleague, working at the Paddington Clinic, suggested I apply for the job there in child psychiatry. This was a decisive step down from QEH, which was closely linked with Great Ormond Street and carried the appointment as teacher at London University. However, I joined the clinic which was then, and never stopped being, trouble ridden; its day hospital was being investigated for the staff's idiosyncratic approach to the treatment of severely disturbed patients, which was tantamount to neglect. After a lengthy scrutiny, it was closed down. The effect on the clinic as a whole was devastating.

I was also developing a private practice as a psycho-analyst. My consulting room was, and still is, in my home, which made it possible to see patients early mornings and evenings, and also gave me a chance to be with the children between appointments. My timetable left little opportunity for relaxing with my family beside weekends. Looking back, the question often arises whether the additional, and sometimes excessive, pressure had hastened the illness by cumulative stress. There was great satisfaction in working in my second and chosen profession and enjoyment in applying the years of strenuous training. The compulsion to work was justified by the need to provide for the children's education, and their relatively young ages made it vital that I continue to work for many years to come. It may stem also from the Parkinsonian personality, which I understood more clearly in later years after concentrated observation and research into the personality of PD sufferers before the onset of their illness. Certainly Parkinsonians can work harder and longer than they are often given to suppose and benefit from it. Motivation to work injects a powerful incentive to well-being, and it was clear to me that disruption of regular schedules by Christmas, Easter and summer holidays wreaked havoc with my stability.

At times I felt an awareness of my decline and in consequence a deadening of sensitivity. The disease was still confined to the left side, with a less firm grip in the hand and some loss of power. I also felt some rigidity in the neck. For a few years I turned a blind eye to any indication that it might be moving over to the right side. I was trying to puzzle out why my illness should be confined to the left side only, and began to have vague thoughts about a psychosomatic link to depression and early object loss. The question in my mind was, if so, would it be reversible?

This half-body illness led me to speculation about the work of Ornstein and Sperry, who were drawing attention at that time to the contrast in function of the left side and the right side of the brain. I was hopeful that the dominance of the left side of the brain might be released by resolving deep conflicts; that the right, feeling-related side centering on time and space, might come to dominate the left with its resources of language and calculation.

Parkinson's disease was, until recent years, still thought of as an old person's disease, and most people were amazed to learn that mine had been diagnosed before I was forty.

There was a post-influenza version of the illness, better recognized and brought to wider notice by Oliver Sacks. It was while talking about his book *Awakenings* on television that Oliver Sacks first came to my attention. In it he describes his treatment of long-hospitalized patients in a nursing home in New York state. They had been suffering from encephalitic PD resulting from the influenza epidemic that raged across the world in 1918. He had brought them out of their Sleeping Beauty state (later dramatized by Harold Pinter in the play *A Kind of Alaska*) to come alive as personalities and be mobile again. It was as if a mysterious barrier had been breached by the use of L-dopa and the excitement generated by this response was beautifully conveyed by Sacks.

I telephoned him when I heard that he was visiting England and explained that I had recently started taking L-dopa and that I would value discussing this with him. He came for supper a few days later, and I was struck by the benign, bear-like quality of the man, particularly the moulded earth boots which made him look poised on hind paws. His vast beard and spectacles gave emphasis to his intellectual qualities which emerged in the conversation. Over a salmon supper, he said that we should keep in touch, which we did indirectly, when I was asked by *The Lancet* to review his autobiographical book *A Leg to Stand On*.

What we had in common was a personal involvement in psychoanalysis and an interest in L-dopa, forming a kind of neuro-psychological mafia. He embodied for me the magical omnipotent effect of L-dopa, and his patients represented the end point of a spectrum of severity, a spectrum which at that time I was just beginning to traverse.

My form of PD was the idiopathic type, that of unknown origin, which affects younger Parkinsonians with greater frequency than those post-encephalitic cases described by Sacks, or those cases resulting from vascular disease in old age. Parkinson's disease can be induced in young people by drugs. Two prominent drugs which can cause this are the major tranquillizer, Phenothiazine (Largactil), and MPTP, a by-product of designer-made heroin.

The finding of the compound MPTP, that can selectively destroy striatal cells in primates and replicate the clinical as well as pathologic state of PD, has given investigators a model in which to study the mechanism of the disease.

A whole cluster of events came together at this time, four years into the illness, to produce a dramatic change in my state. It could be that the inner drama, which had to do with the recognition of my illness, was in search of expression. I couldn't keep quiet about it any longer and I couldn't continue to store it in the recesses of my mind.

Plugged with a constant supply of Sinemet, I had controlled and concealed the tremor and the anxiety, but had paid the price with rigidity, a dyskinetic state and an awful yawning fatigue. There had been five years of that 'sometime state', combined with the feeling of sitting on a time-bomb. I confused my personal experience of negative feelings with nihilism in my role as psychoanalyst. However, I attended an international conference on family therapy in Regents Park and encountered stimulating ideas, especially that of the therapist emerging from behind the couch and getting away from the constraints of one-to-one therapy.

A particularly acute feeling of personal helplessness, at this time, was caused by the death of a senior colleague whom I had approached for therapy following Dr Rubinstein's death. I had known him as a supervisor and found him to be an admirable teacher. Lady Bracknell in Oscar Wilde's *The Importance of Being Earnest* reminds one that: 'To lose one parent, may be regarded as a misfortune, to lose both looks like carelessness'. Since first approaching therapy, soon after coming to England from South Africa in 1954, I have experienced the loss by death of four therapists. The pain and sadness of my previous experience of death has been described in a previous chapter. I tended to blame myself for carelessness.

My neurologist's permanent departure for America had struck a further chord of loss in me, and my first appointment with his successor at the Hammersmith Hospital made things worse. He was a pharmacologist rather than a neurologist and I disapproved of his piecemeal approach to my symptoms, his failure to treat me as a total person and his prescribing additional drugs for symptoms produced by other drugs.

From moods of hopelessness, I swung to therapeutic ardour. This newly found positive interest came to a head in the course of treating a thirteen-year-old girl who had a hysterical paralysis of her left leg following orthopaedic treatment. She was brought to the Paddington Centre for Psychotherapy twice weekly and was carried up the stairs to my room by the ambulance men.

One Friday in July, during her session, I supported her, in the course of our discussion, in walking a few steps. She ended up walking across the room unaided and was able to maintain this ability when I saw her during the following sessions. Along with the physical support, we had discussed together traumatic events of her childhood which had been exacerbated by her entry into puberty – the paralysis represented a compromise solution to her conflicts. In my own mind, this achievement opened up the possibility that the shift might well apply to my 'paralysis', even though it was of a different order.

That Tuesday, I made the decision to stop taking my medication and free myself of its tyranny, taking on my shoulders the responsibility of integrating the physical and the psychological elements. I was excited by the thought that PD might, in my case also, have its genesis in early traumatic emotional experience.

All of a sudden, the draggy, depressed feeling lifted, and hope of hypomanic proportions began to reveal itself with leaving off the drug. After four drug-free days, I became highly excitable. I was unable to sleep, and had flights of ideas. I justified my action because I felt I understood that there was a psychosomatic link between my PD and deep-set depression and, therefore, I hoped I would be capable of resolving it on my own. I had not informed my wife of my intention. By the second day, and after two sleepless nights she became increasingly alarmed and puzzled by my feverish excitement. I pleaded with her not to interfere with the experiment, feeling sure that I would be able to cure myself, as I had my patient. I must have been so convincing, and she so trusting; or my hypomania so contagious and my hopes of curing myself so high, that she joined me in a sort of *folie à deux*. Following a rare drift into sleep I dreamed I gave birth to myself – a symbol of omnipotence and the renewed wish to make myself totally free and independent. My fantasies carried me into untold successes, not the least of which was driving myself in a XJ 120 Jaguar.

I was able, through sheer professional training and experience, to carry on with my work at the clinic that day and the next. But inevitably, the brakes were off. My secretary, a warm and motherly lady, phoned my wife and indicated it would be a good idea to drive me home. In the afternoon, the whole family went to the sports grounds in North London to attend the annual cricket match of their prep. school.

On the fourth day I found myself so excessively excited, and exhausted, that I allowed my wife to call my trusted colleague and friend, Janet Humphrey. When she heard I had not slept for four nights, she saw the glaring signals and ordered my wife to get medical help immediately. Our GP responded quickly to her call. He was puzzled by my condition not being aware that sudden withdrawal of large doses of L-Dopa could bring about such a state; nor did the consultant at the Hammersmith Hospital whom my wife had telephoned, concede any connection. So, fearing that any other sedative might mask the symptoms of brain tumour, he prescribed Largactil, which he brought in his case and left with me to take.

I was familiar with this drug and had used it extensively on young schizophrenic patients in my work as a psychiatric resident in New York in 1962. Unfortunately, our GP was unaware at this time that Largactil would further decrease the neuroreceptors' ability to utilize L-dopa. I deliberated for a while after his departure on whether or not to take it. I just wanted to sleep and hoped for a sedative. But I decided to cooperate and waited as the effects came on, feeling more immobile and losing the sense of my body outline.

I remember feeling I had shrunk into a pathetic infant, crouched in the corner of a dark room, and that I was climbing into my brain. I asked my wife not to leave me. Meantime the consultant psychiatrist at the Royal Free Hospital was called. Although it was Saturday he came to the house and organized a private room for me and, in a near-comatose state from the Largactil, I was helped into our GP's car and with my wife was driven to the hospital.

The hospital at that time was relatively new and as I emerged from the coma-like depths, I felt comfortable there in my own peaceful room with lovely views over Hampstead. All scans and tests confirmed that no organic factors were involved and that time and resumption of my L-dopa was all that was required.

When I recovered from the effects of the trauma, I felt I had committed myself to the strategy of not taking drugs and wanted to see it through as far as possible. The staff, puzzled by the whole episode, seemed willing to leave me be.

After two days of sleeping off the combined effects of the drugs and the hysteria, I woke up at 4 a.m. and looking for something to write on, found a wad of paper used for patient observation. I proceeded to write and to write and to write page after page of an integrated theory of human behaviour. It covered the origins of human emotion, as reflected in behaviour, and looked at the therapeutic relationship in psychotherapy. I made a plea for the facilitation of the patient's development in preference to forcing him into a regressed mode, and stressed the patient's positive functioning aspects which need constantly to be acknowledged in treatments. The idea of eye contact became important. This, as well as recognition of the person, can be lost on the couch. I grappled with survival, the avoidance of excessive pain, loneliness and the helplessness of separateness and independent existence. Finally I found myself writing about the circularity of life with death at the end, and ending as part of the beginning. It was a catharsis.

The psychiatrist in charge, under whom I had worked as a registrar, felt that Lithium was indicated for the hypomania. But I refused to take it, hiding it under my tongue and spitting it out when the dispensing nurse was gone. After that, apart from urging me to take the Sinemet, they let me be and the ward round soon studiously avoided my room. They allowed me to join in swimming and physiotherapy, where my spectacles were smashed in a volley ball exercise, leaving me short-sighted and relishing the new vision which fitted in well with my emotional new vision.

While I had succeeded in overcoming my depression and bringing some understanding to my attitude to myself, no change was yet to be seen in the PD during my drug-free state. I was able to relax the tremor away, but it was heightened whenever a doctor or external observer appeared. I felt I was on the right track, even though a slight tremor and some rigidity persisted. My mood was now calmer and my thinking very clear and unfettered by drugs.

The summer passed with frequent visitors, old friends and new, and colleagues. Our children were a great boost to me, whether in their visiting or the drawings and messages they sent; especially my oldest son, Gideon, aged nine, who was recording in daft cartoons events surrounding my hospital existence, real or imagined. They seemed unaware of the drama being played out around them and felt only the excitement, novel events and their end-of-term sports and social activities, which reminded me of the more devastating drama of my childhood – only in this one, the parent re-emerged from the hospital.

I read avidly. It was the hottest spell this country had known and was followed by the worst floods in the history of north London. I was due to leave the hospital on the day following the drenching. I found the basement of my home soaking from the floods which had penetrated the side door. In the state I was in, I felt identified with the powerful forces of nature that had been unleashed at that moment in time.

The family had survived on the strength and love of my wife, aided by a friend from New York, Ruth Werthman, who was visiting and stayed on to help with organizing the children, leaving Lili to spend long hours with me.

In retrospect, my reaction to the illness, once the quiet defensive denial had proved inadequate, became a hysterical one, based on raw fear. I still was holding on to an idealized image of my body in motion, despite increasing immobility and depression as a consequence of the PD.

An attempt to regress might have seemed preferable to facing the dismal future: a good cry might have produced some relief, yet it seemed that the very nature of the illness inhibited emotional release.

After recovery in hospital, I gave up my bid for self-cure and, behind it, the theory modelled on hysteria and regression. If early emotional traumas were precursors of this neurological disorder, my experience, instead of reversing it, left it unchanged. Years later I was to learn about a more convincing theory when I read Joyce McDougall, a psychoanalyst working in Paris, who has written extensively on psychosomatic conditions. She came to the conclusion that 'all cases of physical damage or ill health in which psychological factors play an important role, are related to psychosomatic phenomena. These include accident-proneness or the lowering of the immunological shield when under stress, so that one falls victim more readily to infectious disease . . . and problems of addiction, which are a "psychosomatic" attempt to deal with distressful conflicts by temporarily blurring an awareness of their existence'. Studying the work of physicians dealing with the psychosomatic illness of babyhood enabled her to understand that her adult patients at certain times function psychically like infants (from the Latin *infans,* meaning one that cannot speak). Since babies cannot yet use words with which to think, they respond to emotional pain only psychosomatically. Although mothers think within a code of language (and most mothers talk constantly to their babies) the infant's earliest psychic structures are built around nonverbal signifiers in which body functions and the erogenous zones play a predominant role. McDougall is not surprised when a baby, who has been suddenly separated from its mother for a long period of time or has been subjected to sudden shock, reacts with gastric hyperfunction or colitis. When an adult constantly does the same thing in similar circumstances resulting in serious illness, McDougall is tempted to conclude that 'we are dealing with an arachaic form of mental functioning that does not use language'. I thought that my predisposition to PD might have had its origins in such an archaic mind-body experience.

A pattern of getting myself taken into hospital in the face of a crisis was now established and was to be repeated later on in Spain and subsequently, Birmingham, where I would be among the early subjects in a pioneering operation. These would also have unconscious links, coming as they did, with psychoanalytic holidays which drove me to seek some replacement refuge.

The holiday came to an end, and the demands of life and work resumed. I went back to low doses of Sinemet and returned to my patients. New zeal as a therapist seemed to emerge from the strait-jacket of my former training, alongside my experience of illness. I was able to treat my patients in a more active and participating way.

Dr Gerald Stern, consultant neurologist at University College Hospital, was contacted and an appointment made for me to see him after I was discharged from the Royal Free

Hospital, where I had been under the care of P.K. Thomas. This was the beginning of a long-lasting contact which was to have some surprising and bizarre moments in the future.

The discharge from hospital left me with much more hope that research would produce something worthwhile, a supplement to L-dopa, and I was going to see what energy I could muster to meet people in the field who I could persuade to hasten the process. At the same time, I would carry on my exploration of the psyche and soma (body) and other aspects of psychotherapy, expressed in my ambitious search for an integrated theory of human behaviour. The work I did, looked at now, contains some highly imaginative creative writing. It was a big step from the initials I designed with a ruler on the blank tile.

CHAPTER 7

The Long Haul:
Trials and Failed Cures

A few months before my breakdown I had read Ernest Hartmann's *Functions of Sleep* in an attempt to understand my feelings of depression, and later of excitement, under the influence of excessive L-dopa.

In this book, Hartmann contrasts D (dream sleep) with S (non-dream sleep), and states that dream sleep has a role in restoring and reorganizing brain catecholamines which include noradrenaline and dopamine. Animal studies showed several functions for brain catecholamines (neuro-transmitters), including control of motor activity in the corpus striatum (that part of the brain where the loss of cells produces PD). These brain amines also play an important part in the higher function of the brain, the cortex.

Hartmann was impressed clinically by the ability of dexteramphetamine (a cerebral stimulant) in mimicking catecholamines to produce a state of increased energy resembling hypomania, when first administered. He showed that the patient becomes compulsive if too much is taken, and paranoid if the amount is further increased. When the drug is withdrawn, a severe clinical depression is likely. Catecholamines energize the four 'f's, – fight, flight, food and sexual behaviour (Pribram). Most important, however, is that all these psychological states can be reproduced by alteration in brain catecholamines functioning in relatively normal individuals. A predisposition to illness is not required to account for these effects. In the same way, dopamine excess can produce a similar sequence of behaviours. When dopamine is stopped, depression is produced, especially when the receptors have been used to overstimulation by excesses of dopamine.

I was failing to note that dopamine, with all its potential qualities, acted differently at receptors in the corpus striatum from those in the cortical network involved with sleep and dreams. What I did observe, however, is that when taking large doses of L-dopa, the effect would be beyond that desired and would produce effects on sleep as well as causing psychosis and hallucination. These symptoms would diminish as the dose was lowered.

At Hampstead Clinic I was part of a research group looking at early manifestations of anxiety in children. We focused on pre-oedipal (birth to two years) anxiety resulting from disturbance in the mother-child relationship. This influenced my thoughts that my own anxiety had originated well before my mother's death, and favoured my view of the persistence of an early split between mind and body which later gave rise to the anxiety-tremor. I was trying to pull together these elements but with hindsight, the truth, which I was trying to deny, was that although anxiety may have made the tremor worse, the tremor had a life of its own, independent of the body's reaction to it or the context in which it occurred. The magical feeling that I had complete control over my body in all situations obscured my true helplessness. It also lent itself to a continuing search for psychological elements from my infancy that I hoped would be unravelled with new insight, and be of benefit to me. As the illness shifted to involve the right side of the body, and its severity increased, this approach became less supportable.

The inability to move, at times, and the helplessness that accompanies it, were best faced in their own right, instead of being associated with a feeling of guilt that I myself was responsible for the illness, whether held in or projected outwards. This too is less pronounced as the years progress. In my mind, my work had been confused with my illness, to the detriment of both, and I realized that to resolve this confusion I would require further self-analysis after completion of my formal training analysis.

Hartmann's main hypothesis is that the findings of psychoanalysis and those of academic psychology have a common basis in behaviour, and in the everyday reality of life, mind and body were not split, but were rather ways of reading and understanding complementary data. There is no mysterious leap or mind-body gap between the physiological-chemical description and the psychological description of the underlying process. The gap or leap exists only between the subjective experience and the underlying process. Psychoanalysis does concern itself with subjective meaning in a way often avoided by academic psychology.

My enthusiasm and greater awareness of the deep ramifications of the treatment relationship, communicated itself to my psychotherapy and analytic patients. They responded to it and to the illustration of that interaction. There was a creative area of play and exploration between patient and therapist in which trust and self-esteem could be rebuilt. Winnicott, the eminent paediatrician and psycho-analyst, had drawn attention to this significance which had struck him, coming as he did from a background of paediatrics and psychoanalysis. To him, the quality of the mother-child relationship was the foundation of all subse-quent relationships.

I had freed myself from the doctrinaire reliance on classical psychoanalytic theory and moved to a maverick position in which my own individuality did not have to be supressed, but rather could be harnessed in support of the interaction with the patient. This had to be achieved without subduing the patient's assertiveness, which was better for the ultimate reconciliation of the loving and hating capacity of the patient and the elimination of splits between these two. Technically this was made possible by the umbrella support offered to the patient's self-esteem on the one hand, while exploring conflicts and losses and deficiencies on the other hand. By active and directed work in this area, I found that treatment was speeded up, and better results obtained.

While I was formulating these concepts new neurochem-icals were emerging for use in research of Parkinson's disease.

Deprenyl
At this time, living back to back with us in our new home in St Johns Wood, was a most interesting retired scientist, who had made his name and fortune in the development of the heart-lung machine. A Hungarian with a peremptory voice and a heavy limp from a wartime adventure, he was always ready to show an interest in ideas. More importantly, he knew how to activate them.

I read in *The Times* that a biochemist in Hungary had

developed a chemical which acts to inhibit the oxidation (burning up) of brain chemicals, a so-called monoamine-oxidase inhibitor. This did not have the dangerous reaction to such products as cheese that other MAOs had when given to depressed patients. It was taken up by Birkmayer in Vienna for use in trials on Parkinson's disease. Prof. Birkmayer was an early pioneer with Hornikiewicz in the application of large doses of L-dopa and was later to figure in my search for a cure. During one of our regular luncheons that we enjoyed together, my Hungarian friend was interested to hear the news and said that he would phone Budapest where he had strong and reliable connections. Not long afterwards, he delivered personally over the garden fence, a small phial containing little yellow pills. Dr Stern was about to do a therapeutic trial of the same drug, and I was pleased to join in. I subsequently had doubts about it, but have continued to take it, with some interruption, for thirteen years. Current research indicates that it has a delaying effect on the continuing deterioration of the disease.

Endorphins

A good deal of excitement was being generated by the discovery of encephalins by Prof. Hans Kosterlitz in Edinburgh. He came to lunch at my house in May 1978 and discussed his work which had uncovered the body's own ability to produce pain-killers in the form of opiates. I thought that as modulators of catacholamines, the endorphin might act as a fine tuner to the L-dopa response. I thought it possible that the repressed pain of loss might be acting through thought-inhibiting pathways in the brain at a higher level.

The field of peptide research was emerging with similar promise. Prof. de Wied, in Utrecht, was a pioneer, and I corresponded with him and visited him in his laboratory in

Holland. He was warm and enthusiastic, but didn't feel he had much to offer. We agreed to remain in touch and he subsequently tried out on me an Organon peptide drug, developed for pain response. But it didn't have any effect on the modulation of the L-dopa and left the capricious On-Off, the functioning or non-functioning of the medication, unaffected.

The theory I was working on seemed to be more and more shaky. Then the news broke of the use of Beta-endorphins, synthesized by a chemist in San Francisco. This had been given to schizophrenics by Nathan Kline, an experienced organic psychiatrist, working at the Rockland Hospital in New York state. When I telephoned him there, he said he only had a sufficient supply of Beta-endorphin for his patients and could spare me none.

Thus ended my exploration of a trail that had turned out to lead nowhere. I had embarked on this following a hunch which had turned out to be incorrect, namely that dopamine was a neurotransmitter common to both schizophrenia and Parkinson's disease. Despite it being in excess in schizophrenia and deficient in Parkinson's disease, there appears to be no correlation between the two illnesses.

CHAPTER 8

The Middle Years

I had been corresponding with neurologists and psychoanalysts in the United States and felt it a good time to follow up letters with personal meetings. In 1979 the opportunity came to exchange houses in the summer with an American family on Cape Cod. The house, in which we were to spend the summer, was in an enchanted wood in Brewster and belonged to an eminent naturalist. Even the spiders in the home were safeguarded, with instructions pinned on little notes that they were not to be touched.

For the first week, because we had left our driving licences at home, we walked everywhere except when given lifts. Walking in file, all five of us, on the side of the cars-only roads, presented a strange sight to the car-bound populus of the Cape. We got to know the roads pebble by pebble. We were taken into the highly articulate, somewhat eccentric, society of retired artists, writers, film directors and musicians, who colonized the area. We moved in a wide and hospitable circle with daily cocktail parties, dinners, barbecues and clambakes on the magnificent beaches. I greatly enjoyed diving into the high breakers. Not only the people, but the flora and fauna, became familiar through the guidance from afar of our host, John Hay, who was meantime exploring the landscaped plots of gardens in St John's Wood.

At the end of the summer we went to New York, where I spoke to Roger Duvoisin, a leading neurologist at Mount Sinai Hospital, who had published a study on twins, from which he deduced that PD was not hereditary. This tallied with my preoccupation that the origins of the disease in at least a group of PD sufferers were in early childhood.

Our last stop-off was to the National Institute of Health at Bethesda. This is the seat of American research, a vast, sprawling complex in a suburb of Washington DC, where some of the best brains from Britain and the world have been attracted to participate in their research. I had left my family in the car park, and went to keep my appointment with Donald Calne. We talked of my pet theories about PD as a manifestation of deep endogenous depression. He was interested, but I recognized that his pursuit of drugs that would improve the physical, and indirectly, the emotional condition of patients who consulted him and thousands of others, was more productive.

From talking to Parkinson's disease patients who were referred to me, I would have to admit that understanding their background may do no more than relieve some of the self-hatred felt by many sufferers. Despairing in their urgent need to find an explanation for this mysterious illness, they blame themselves for their decline, yet find themselves unable to reverse the situation. This understanding might well be useful in the early stages of the illness. It requires a degree of emotional maturity to cope with the altering body image that is part and parcel of the Parkinsonian predicament and to retain some feeling of control over the situation.

I was still trying to understand my illness using psychoanalytic concepts, interweaving them with ideas culled from neurobiology. Parkinsonians would notice considerable variation in response to L-dopa according to their mood; this interaction of drugs and mood remains something of a paradox and a mystery and may only become clearer with a better understanding of the emotional developmental history of a particular patient. In this way the broad dimensions of Parkinson's disease might be understood.

An important question is whether the growing immobility seen in the illness produces personality changes, or whether these merely indicate the personality of the Parkinsonian before the onset of his illness. In my view, deep-set depression is present in the make-up of many PD sufferers, especially in the early onset under-forties group. To defend against the emotional pain and depression, most sufferers employ a defensive device termed 'operational thinking'. An example is given by Joyce McDougall. She quotes a patient who, when faced with the tragedy of having run over a pedestrian and asked whether she was upset, responded that she wasn't because she was insured against accidents. Such people restrict their relationships to the isolated functions of people rather than relating them to the whole person.

The fundamental fears of the operational thinker are of disintegrating and falling into total helplessness. They appear to show a deadening of ordinary response early on in life and a heightened activation in subsequent crises. What are taken as ordinary problems by some, become life and death crises for future Parkinsonians. There is a deadening of fine feeling and a subsequent loss of subtlety of action, producing reality-bound patients. The ordinary exchanges that nurture emotional development may, as a result of overwhelming experiences, like death or failure to mourn, lose their ordinary flexibility and become rigid. What gets suppressed is the personal imagination and with it an ability to relate to others. Guilt and responsibility are controlled in this way. Winnicott reminds us of a reactive 'false self' personality with a depressive core living in constant fear of breakdown.

This is particularly problematic with the On-Off, which comes into prominence three to five times a day after the beginning of treatment and occurs a number of times daily. When Off, one shuffles with the *petit pas*, characteristic of Parkinson's disease, and finds it difficult to navigate oneself in a crowd because the righting reflexes have failed and one feels clumsy. When On, one's body expands, the rhythm is restored and for the span of its efficacy, one is tricked into feeling normal and even athletic and that it will last.

The On-Off is, without doubt, central in importance to patients with chronic Parkinsonism. One needs to be On to meet friends, discuss issues, participate spontaneously in social activities, deal with family crises and, in my case, see patients and work. Dealing with any problem without benefit of drugs exposes one as reticent and lacking in confidence, which is difficult to cover up. Drops at the end of a dose could be adjusted by careful timing to avoid lags in the relay and ensure continuity. But as the illness progresses, there are unaccounted for drops in mid-dose that add complications. Other drugs have become available to tide over these drops, but are not always successful.

L-dopa is quite unique as a drug. Its mode of action does not allow for the continuity of action expected from most other drugs. It is difficult enough to maintain a consistent blood-level bearing in mind the vicissitudes of digestion and absorption. Even if these are optimal, the beneficial effects of the drug are limited to certain hours, which decrease as the illness progresses.

The strength and mobility available during the On periods may be used for self-help physical activities and psychotherapy. The On periods help to make a patient feel integrated for at least part of the time. The Off period, in contrast, is depressing and a reminder of failure. When On, the patient doesn't necessarily feel he needs help; when Off, help would be useless and besides he feels physically unable to make use of such help. A further reason for the neglect of psychotherapy lies in the all or nothing attitude of the neurologist to the illness which is seen as wholly organic rather than on a psychosomatic spectrum. *All* Parkinsonians are menaced by both real and neurotic threats to their equilibrium; the first, because of organic damage, the latter, because old instinctual conflicts to do with the body are revived by the illness – the appearance of earlier patterns of shyness, self-consciousness and sexual withdrawal.

Still trying to reconcile psychoanalysis and neurobiology, as I experienced it as part of PD, I contacted Nathan Kline before taking the plane home from America. He promised to send some Beta-endorphin to London to Prof. Linford-Rees, at that time president of the Royal College of Psychiatry. This sought-after drug never arrived. But through this encounter I came across Prof. Watson whose work on bio-feedback had earlier excited my interest.

Bio-feedback is a self-help device in which a patient responds to a cue given by a machine which then alters again, once the stimulus has been adequately handled. It can be used for patients with any condition in which relaxation is a desired goal. I sat in a dark room at St Bart's under the guidance of Prof. Watson's technician and was so observant of the rules, straining to handle an electric light stimulus, that I produced a retinal tear. I came home with blurred vision in one eye and spent the evening at the outpatients' department at the opthalmic hospital in Marylebone, wondering if I would fully regain my sight. Fortunately after some days, my vision restored itself, and bio-feedback gave way to a venture into acupuncture.

A colleague at the Hampstead Clinic lent me a book by Felix Mann called *Acupuncture, the Cure of Many Diseases*. This ancient Chinese treatment consists of inserting thin needles into strategic nerve points on the body's surface. These send impulses to the diseased part of the body to correct the malady through the subconscious part of the nervous system.

A friend recommended a practitioner, and twice a week I went dutifully up the hill to a Georgian house in Highgate. I couldn't have fed my scepticism a more succulent morsel. As I lay on the hard bed and watched him jiggling around on my skin, I thought, 'Todes, you're really nuts!' Nevertheless, because I assumed the man's professionalism and had committed myself to a trial, I persevered, coming home flushed, tired and hopeful. Until one day, a designer friend of my wife casually mentioned that my acupuncturist was known to her as a designer, well known in the furniture business. This disqualified him in my eyes and I stopped going up that hill.

One further step into alternative medicine took me into the world of the spirit. I did it to please a close friend who knew somebody who claimed success with electrical forces in his hands. I agreed to an assignation in the home of the British Spiritualist Society's splendidly seedy headquarters in Belgrave Square, benignly watched over by the ghosts of Sir Arthur Conan Doyle and Sir Oliver Lodge, the two most renowned leaders of the cult in their day. If I was expecting to be met by Sherlock Holmes, I was disappointed when fetched from the waiting room by a heavily perfumed and bejewelled ship owner who was moonlighting as a layer-on of non-medical hands. He was warm and concerned until he lost his temper with my inability to control my tremor.

Watching the proceedings was a trainee spiritualist. I hope she gained more from the experience than I did. When during the session my drug came On, my 'healer' felt it was completely of his own doing and his treatment vindicated. I walked outside, grateful for the fresh air and that there had been no witnesses that I knew.

For a brief while, I flirted with the idea that eliminating dietary allergens could relieve PD symptoms. An Australian physician in Perth had had some good results with patients by this means. The idea was to clear the system by restricting food to rice and pears and then after two weeks to offer various foods, one at a time, as a challenge to ascertain the response.

My gourmet instincts felt badly bruised after a week of this regime and I reverted to everyday poisons without testing the theory.

The final elements to the Beta-endorphin story were enacted at Guy's Hospital and later UCH, where I was given intravenous injections of the substance sent by de Wied. But as there was no blood-chemistry analysis yet available, it was put into the freezer to await assessment. Clinically, nothing significant happened. I went on with my Sinemet, still troubled with end-of-dose wearing off, mid-point dyskinesia and no smoothing of the transition from one dose to another. This applied as well to the doses of a similar order given at UCH.

Through Prof. Roy Spector at Guy's I got in touch with David Parkes at King's College Hospital who seemed more willing to explore new directions.

Bromocriptine had emerged as a dopamine agonist (reinforcing the action of dopamine) which acted upon the synapse or neural junction in a more prolonged way – if less intensely. The side effect was that it could readily precipitate psychosis in susceptible individuals. After my experience with the withdrawal of L-dopa, I was in no hurry to risk it. However, new agonists were about to be tried and I volunteered for their use on me. Although I was mobile and experiencing only a minor handicap I remained fearful of the future and possible deterioration. I still felt the clock was against me. I had an intravenous dose of Lisuride from Dr Parkes, which made the hairs on my neck bristle but did not produce an On-like state as did L-dopa. I kept in touch with Dr Parkes, who was much more accessible as he was employed full-time.

I returned to the care of Dr Stern and his senior registrar, Dr Lees, for a trial of Pergolide. This too was an agonist, which, it was hoped, might replace L-dopa, especially if used intravenously to achieve steady blood-levels. Because L-dopa requires large quantities of saline to make it soluble when injected into the bloodstream, it was hoped that Pergolide, being readily soluble, might achieve all the effects L-dopa did. This was not to be.

I was now in touch with UCH and King's, the two hospitals which led the field in Parkinson's research. I felt a bit like a go-between. At King's, I took part in a study of intravenous L-dopa which showed that if one could get around the absorption problem, one would eliminate some of the fluctuations in response to the drug. This study conducted by Niall Quinn was an important one, and though with no immediate clinical spin-off, given the right chemical, intravenous delivery would bypass the liver and become more rapidly effective. The principle was to be used in subsequent work with Lisuride.

In 1979 we exchanged homes with an Israeli couple, to be in the centre of Jerusalem. We spent some weeks touring the country, visiting friends and historical sites. We included a visit to Prof. Youdim, who had done much of the early clinical work on Deprenyl and was very enthusiastic. I saw him in his laboratory at his clinic in Haifa, which had magnificent views over the bay.

I went into University College Hospital at Christmas time in 1981, wearing an electronic monitor while starting on small doses of Pergolide. These were gradually increased and I felt some support in the background. I subsequently continued with Pergolide for a number of years, noting that it boosted libido. It also tended to promote breast development.

The following year, Dr Parkes mentioned that he was going to South Africa to lecture on Parkinson's disease. I thought it would be a good opportunity to put together some thoughts on a personal view about the disease by a psychiatrist, and arranged to join him there. I was invited to give my lecture at the academic psychiatric hospital at Tara where Dr Feldman was professor. It was well received and I stayed with my sister and her family, having time to explore places familiar from my childhood. The house in which I was born and grew up was barely recognizable, the brickwork now covered with stucco, and the leaded light windows replaced by large panes of glass. I visited the cemeteries where my parents are buried and thought about my mother's funeral that I hadn't been allowed to attend. I found myself able to shed tears by her grave forty years on. How different my life might have been, I thought for the hundredth time, had antibiotics been available in 1938. Very likely I would have had no need to enter the helping profession or better still, I would have been free to do so without compulsion.

The lecture was the basis of a subsequent paper in *The Lancet* on the same subject and in a way, a forerunner to this book. It was translated and reprinted in a number of languages. It also put me in touch with Parkinsonians from all over the world, some of whom I still correspond with. The knowledge that someone else beside themselves is familiar with their struggle has given reassurance to many in the dismal hours of depression and there was a large response, not only from sufferers, but their families too. The article put into words thoughts and feelings they were experiencing but were not able to express.

I appeared in a film in 1983 entitled *One lives one's life the best one can*. A company was commissioned by Roche Products to make a video film showing recent developments in Parkinson's disease to inform GPs about the social and psychological problems of Parkinson's patients. They enlisted the support and participation of Prof. Marsden, as well as an experienced GP in this field, together with one of his patients. I was interviewed in my home descending the staircase to start the day in my consulting room. I was also filmed playing indoor tennis and handling ceramic pots I had made.

The film rambled on without direction after a good opening on framed graphics. I was grievously overdosed, full of grimaces and postures. To my embarrassment, its showing was not limited, as promised, to the medical profession. It seemed to me that it accomplished little and missed an excellent opportunity to instruct.

CHAPTER 9

Pamplona

In 1982, The Paddington Centre, with its history of conflict and staff difficulties, moved premises from Harrow Road to a new venue. Lancaster Grove was a few steps from the Portobello Road and it was a great relief to move from an atmosphere of concrete flyovers and an endless flow of heavy traffic, to one of overripe fruit and a constant bustle of people in the market. It was also the crossroads and centre of the drug trade with a lot of police attention. The move brought with it a liveliness that was appreciated by all.

My work consisted of assessing the children referred to me, on their own and within their family, and directing them to individual, family, or group therapy. Some came to me for brief therapeutic intervention and I supervised junior staff and clinic associates working with children and their parents. In the community, I was involved with regular weekly groups of health visitors, supervised school medical officers, and worked with GPs in the area on the psychosomatic problems of children. I led, and participated in, large groups of community workers which was very rewarding. I also consulted at local children's nurseries, dealing with developmental problems and abuse.

Committees proliferated at this time of retrenchment in the NHS with its climate of political manipulation; there was talk of closure or merger. In the early to middle 1980s, the staff felt constantly threatened. After every vacation, one was never quite sure whether there was a clinic, or a job, to come back to. A number of senior colleagues and good friends of mine took early retirement and moved out.

By this time, fourteen years into the illness, I was affected on both sides of the body and experienced difficulty in speaking in large groups. I found that by the time I was ready and on the point of saying my bit, the talk had moved on to a new topic. So I confined myself to small groups, diagnostic assessments, supervisions and one-to-one treatment of patients. The notion of not being active and sharing my experience was tantamount to being incommunicado, and I intended to fight off this state with all the energy I had left. I felt I had something to contribute as a person and a physician, even if I had to accommodate certain limitations.

In the autumn of 1985, refreshed by an exceptionally rewarding holiday in Rome, with avid sightseeing including a day-long trip through the Vatican galleries, I returned to work with a will and energy. I mobilized myself to organize my drug in order to obtain maximum continuity.

Demands for leadership in the clinic were coming to a

head, as there was repeated talk of closure and, or, merging of the clinic with a neighbouring one. Unfilled sessions were left unfilled and voluntary redundancies were being sought. I appeared a vulnerable candidate and the pressure on me from my colleagues to resign, on the grounds of ill-health, was mounting. A meeting was convened by the fellow consultants in my clinic, to which they summoned me and told me that my presence at the Paddington Centre was negatively affecting the clinic in its struggle for survival, and that therefore I should resign or submit myself to the scrutiny of the Three Wise Men. This is a body of doctors drawn from a pool of consultants who would make an objective assessment of a doctor's fitness to work.

Wanting to retain my job, in which I felt competent, I in turn put pressure on my doctors, especially Dr Parkes, who was willing to try anything to help. He favoured the use of subcutaneous delivery to resolve the problem of drug continuity. The question was to find a drug without bad side effects which could be delivered in this way. I felt my confidence could be boosted and that I could hold on to my job were this to be successful.

I had a trial of Terguride as an outpatient. It produced vomiting on the side ward and later in the car on the way home. The hospital had thoughtfully provided a kidney-shaped bowl. While making me nauseous, the drug failed to produce an On which I was used to with L-dopa.

Dr Parkes mentioned that a colleague, Dr Obeso, had been experimenting with a subcutaneous pump, an adaptation of one used for diabetics. He had learned his technique during a year attached to the King's College neurology unit. Dr Parkes offered to write to him at Pamplona, northern Spain, where he was continuing his research at the university hospital. To add to the mood for enterprise, Dr Parkes gave me to understand that the drug company, Schering, would underwrite at least some of the expense connected with the experiment, and a good friend of many years generously offered to contribute to the cost.

My enthusiasm when pursuing a new development in the treatment of PD is irresistable, my hopes contagious. My desire to continue working was very strong. I infected not only my family but our lifelong friends in Barcelona, the painter Garcia Llort and his wife, who invited us to stay in their home *en route*. They introduced us to a Catalan neurologist who had checked out the hospital where I was going and the Opus Dei for which it was a flagship and the envy of all institutions of higher learning in Spain. He has a brother with PD and was awaiting the outcome of my trial to enrol him in the same course.

So on a Sunday in early April during the Easter school holidays, my wife, my daughter and I found ourselves on a train to Pamplona. We had spent three days in Barcelona with our friends. As was my habit in preparation for a drug trial, in order to simplify the picture (in fact it often complicates it), I had stopped taking Pergolide and Deprenyl, and was suffering the usual symptoms of withdrawal. It had been heavy going. The good weather was freakishly interrupted by a snow storm two miles out of Pamplona and we arrived at the station after a three-hour journey from Barcelona, to see the town under a cover of white. Nature again was reminding us to be fully prepared for surprises, and not only good ones.

A taxi took us from the station to the hospital, which was impressive. It was a sprawling collection of concrete-faced buildings, it looked like a small community, with its formal gardens, sculpted lawns, a shrine, and, dominating it, a senate house and lodgings for the religious community which ran it. The red-brick medical school fronted the hospital building. The whole complex was situated on the outskirts of Pamplona and one could see the Pyrenees rising out of the Navarro valley.

Inside, the walls were panelled with oak and the mirror-like floors were of marble. The sound of footsteps and especially the high heels of auxiliary staff and the visitors who flooded into the corridors all day long, echoed through the rooms. We checked into the hospital and I was allocated a room on the first floor with an armchair that conveniently converted into a bed and a bathroom attached.

My wife negotiated all the formalities, being fluent in Spanish. A TV faced the bed, but we discovered that programmes were confined mainly to bullfights and religious subjects. I had attended a bullfight on the Costa Brava but disliked a game in which the opponent doesn't know the rules. Over the bed, there was an agonized mawkish effigy of Christ on the Cross. I was reminded of similar votives on the walls of our servants' quarters in Johannesburg as a child. Both gave me a feeling of unease in my stomach. My first hospital meal was far more interesting on first acquaintance than NHS food, but when my wife and daughter left to go to their hotel in town that night and I was left alone, I discovered that English-speaking nurses were a rarity.

On Monday morning, Dr Obeso introduced himself and his team. He had the dark-eyed look of a matinée idol with sleek black hair. He wore a white coat and spoke excellent English. He received the gift we had bought for him with enthusiasm; it was a collage depicting a village cricket match to remind him of his stay in our country.

Briskly and convincingly, he outlined his treatment plan. I said I would like to meet one of the successfully treated patients. His paper in *The Lancet* had claimed twenty-three successes of treatment with the Lisuride infusion. He quite agreed that we should meet his patient Charlie, as well as the doyenne of all his successful achievements, Maria Dolores, a South American woman who had made international headlines with her recovery as a result of this treatment. He mentioned that Prof. Calne would be visiting during the next week and he hoped to have something to show him. He himself would not be available for the coming weekend because he had to attend an international conference in London. He welcomed the charts of my response to my medication, which I had conscientiously kept, and said that Lisuride treatment in minimal dosage would begin on Tuesday.

That afternoon, like a boarder on a precious school holiday, I was allowed out and, with Lili and Ariane, wandered around the old town of Pamplona. We looked at the bullring, lying quiet at this time of the year, and had an ice-cream on the terrace of the Hotel Irun which Hemingway immortalized. The colonnades of the square and the old cathedral, the little alleys where the bulls run to their slaughter, had some charm, even in the wintry bleakness. But going back to the suburbs, there was a stark contrast with avenues lined by supermarkets, banks and modern brick blocks, some of which were being built without scaffolding, the unprotected workers crawling precariously on the concrete blocks.

The hospital served the district and was the end stop of the bus line. Pamplonans are proud of it; it is well funded by the Opus Dei and attracts excellent professional staff because of its modern facilities and reputation throughout Spain.

We now settled into a daily routine. The private phone next to my bed probably saved my sanity. It enabled me to keep in touch with my wife and daughter early each morning at their hotel and tell them my overnight news. They, too, were reassured about my state and arrived in the late morning carrying their lunch of yoghurt and sliced cold meat which they ate with me, together with the remains of mine, in my room. The food quickly became uneatable; the greasy Parmentier omelette, onions and potatoes fried in heavy olive oil was generally cold and made me nervous. My daughter was good company for my wife. If she had craved to be back in London enjoying her school holidays, she never revealed it. Instead, we played scrabble and bridge and awaited events.

CHAPTER 10

The Lisuride Episode

Next day, using Sinemet, they did an assessment of me, noting On and Off periods. I joined my wife and daughter at the end of their lunch in a café outside the hospital. In the afternoon, at 4 o'clock precisely, a woman doctor came to initiate the pump, putting a needle into the subcutaneous tissue of the abdomen on the right side and connecting it to the pump which was the size of an audio casette. I was premedicated with an anti-emetic, Domperidone, not to be confused with the delectable Champagne. I soon fell asleep, reassured by the thought that the game was on the way. When I awoke, there were hints of nausea. That night, I could hardly sleep with excitement. The following day, they arranged to start the pump at one o'clock. I was Off, so I hardly participated in its being placed. The doctor was very adept: the needle was under the skin and joined up to the power source before I knew it.

I decided to keep a diary of the events.

Now that the *bomba* (as it is called) is in place, I've cheered up no end. It seems to boost a faltering level of Sinemet. Before leaving for his weekend journey, Dr Obeso and I had a long talk. I told him of my experience with the Terguride and gathered from him that there was a lot of international interest in his Lisuride experiment; he said that the Germans and the Italians had had some success but some of the King's College subjects had failed because of hallucinations.

Thursday. I was visited by Father Juan, a handsome, olive-skinned priest from Lima, Peru, in the Order of the Opus Dei. He has a brilliant, contagious smile, and a real feeling for humanity. He also speaks good English, and told me about the place of the Opus Dei in the Catholic hierarchy. We arranged to play tennis together.

In the afternoon, I met Lili and Ariane and we went shopping in a department store in the old city. They took me to the Hotel Yoldi, in Art Deco style, in the commercial part of town and showed me their temporary quarters. I felt overdosed and scaled the Sinemet down. This evening, I had a visit from Father David, a Rhodes scholar and Harvard graduate from Rhode Island. He was not subtle about his brief to convert me to his branch of the religion he represented. He could see he was getting courteously nowhere. (He was never to come back again.)

Friday. The pump was working unobtrusively and produced a lot of grimaces and mannered movements in the afternoon. It was supposed to be a good sign that the dopa was in excess and should be reduced, while the Lisuride should be increased. There was no nausea or depersonalization.

Saturday. I have a visit from an undertaker, his wife and daughter, arranged through a nursing sister who took my daughter on an outing. Sunday I seemed to get no benefit. The doctor discovered the needle was blocked and the substance was not penetrating. Later that evening it worked.

Monday. The highlight of the day has been playing tennis with Father Juan. I came On as we stepped onto the court and played for an hour. I found it exhausting. I felt a fraud walking into the hospital with a tennis racquet where people were dying. I went on a tour of the campus taken by the public relations dept of the Opus Dei. The senate building had vast reception rooms and lecture amphitheatres and there was an eerie feeling about those halls, all those portraits and chandeliers and gilt making the place look more like a presidential palace than a university complex. Father Juan visited in the evening and told me he had explained his frequent and welcome visits to his superior by saying that he was improving his English, albeit by speaking with an infidel.

Tuesday. I went for a walk to the old town, looking at the statue of Hemingway outside the bullring and window shopping in the square.

Wednesday. The pace is hotting up. It is like a

74

new shooting match. Obeso came in mid-morning and looked at my carefully maintained charts on graph paper, like a general surveying the front. He coolly pointed out flaws, and went off to deploy his army and arrange a new attack. He dismissed Lili's pressured certainty that the body-nature sometimes needs a rest; that we should accept this limitation. He presented a diametrically opposed view: that it has nothing to do with nature but is a problem of drug and synaptic kinetics. I said I would need to be totally convinced about this and reminded him that the map is not the territory, the graph not the person. He promised that we would meet two of his twenty-two patients next day who were being brought in for Donald Calne's visit. He said he is convinced he is capable of producing an uninterrupted On with patients and could do away with Offs completely.

Having gone shopping to find presents for Ariane's sixteenth birthday and returned exhausted, in strode Charlie! A French Jewish Parkinsonian, one of Obeso's early patients, he comes in for stabilization every few months. From his conversation in French with Lili, we gathered that he arranged these sessions to fit in with the bullfights of which he was an aficionado. He was overdosed, and as he talked, I felt I was looking in a mirror recognizing all my grimaces. His life story and background was troubled. His parents were deportees from Poland; he and his sister hidden by a Catholic family. When reunited with their mother, she could not accept his sister's love affair with a non-Jew, and his sister threw herself under a train in the Paris Métro. He had found a kind of peace, Parkinson's and all, in tax-free

Andorra, where he had gone to settle with his wife and two children.

Thursday. Obeso surprised Dr Calne with me. They had read the clinical notes of my history, and Calne thought that I had done remarkably well over the fourteen years. I noted that he looked a little older and greyer. I said I was hanging on to my job by the skin of my teeth, and hoped that the treatment would give me a new lease of life for both work and leisure. They discussed how my Sinemet dose had been lowered from 0.7 gm to 0.5 gm.

Charlie visited me in the afternoon with Maria Dolores, whom he looks after when they are both brought to Pamplona for viewing by 'visiting firemen'. A slightly built, bent-sideways lady, playing with her choker and smilingly disporting her English, she could walk only from a jump-start and then couldn't stop. On this occasion she was in a wheel chair pushed by Charlie, who displayed her with pride. Charlie came back to play a board game with Ariane and gave her an electronic solar game. He wanted very much to please and would have given everything away to make himself be acceptable. He spoke in a tense, driven way and Lili had a hard time coping with his pressured way of talking. How he can communicate with his trial doctors, knowing only French and Yiddish and they knowing only Spanish, is a mystery. A lot must be based on conjecture.

He was still there when Obeso came, and his frantic talking made it difficult for me to get in a word. This was imperative, because Obeso had decided to increase the dose of Lisuride. We celebrated my daughter's birthday with a delectable confection Lili had ordered from the pastry shop in town, a long *abrazo de gitano* (Gypsy's arm) – a light sponge roll clad in custard and decorated for the occasion. We couldn't finish it, even with the help of the nurses.

Obeso decided to put up the dose of Lisuride next day.

Friday. Had disturbed sleep at the thought of a higher dose and the knowledge that some patients at King's College had experienced severe enough psychosis to terminate the trial of the drug. I was woken in the middle of the night by a bang followed by a drip. I wasn't sure whether I or someone else had caused this noise. I had a strange feeling of words and thoughts being contiguous, as if there was a physical awareness of thought and my body image no longer existed. When I repeated this to Lili in my early morning call to the hotel, alarm bells rang with her and she hurried in to speak with Dr Pastor, the woman doctor, pleading with her not to step up the dose. I waited tensely for Obeso's ward round. He questioned me about my mental state, which I answered in a less professional way than I might, contrasting the image of a quiet side and a wild side in my personality. He made it very clear that limits to Sinemet usage between 0.25 gm and 0.5 gm can only be reduced by using more Lisuride, a total of 2.5 mgm. When later we went down to Dr Pastor in the outpatients' department, we ran into Dr Martinez Lage, the chief of neurology, who was very enthusiastic about the trial.

I went for a walk round the old city, and bought *The Heart of the Matter* by Graham Greene, reflecting that my talks with Father Juan had stirred my interest in Catholicism, and preparing for the weekend departure of Lili. Obeso assured us that there would be no rise in dose over the weekend and that they would look after me while my wife left to take our daughter back to England for the beginning of term.

I heard Obeso was under some pressure to get his results together for presentation at the International Congress the following week in Atlanta Georgia.

I was feeling insecure and more introspective than usual, the strange thought lurking in my mind that an extraordinary experiment was going to take place, a first-time, award-winning performance, and that I might not survive it. In retrospect, I was reacting to being left in hospital on my own, and exposed to psychosis-inducing chemicals.

Sunday. A grey, overcast Sunday. As I was leaving to take my family to the bus terminal for the journey to Bilbao, the door opened and there appeared in a wheel chair a human wreck of a man, completely catatonic. We had heard from Charlie how this silent staring man had been affected by the Lisuride on his return to Morocco and now, back in Pamplona, they were unsuccessfully trying to remedy matters. It was not a reassuring sight.

We took the town bus to the terminal. I was grimacing and felt embarrassed. It was a strange experience walking through the underpass frequented by winos, old, decrepit, injured, cast-offs from society. One man dragging himself legless along the pavement like a snake. I waved goodbye to my family as they got on the bus, and going back through the litter-strewn terminus, I had a deeply depressing feeling, reminiscent of a similar state on Hospital Hill when my mother died. Suddenly, I felt completely lost without the language, and Lili's departure exposed me to terrible fears of not being able to make myself understood. I grabbed the nearest taxi and drove back to the hospital where a welcome sight, Charlie, was waiting to play tennis.

He took me to a club in the outskirts of Pamplona, where he had booked in on the strength of my being a doctor. We played in a bubble, a blown-up tent, proof against the weather. He swung his arm violently and we nearly had a fight when I asked to use my good metal racquet I had brought from England and which he had commandeered. He said he couldn't play without it. Not that he could play with it. He'd made arrangements for a taxi driver to pick us up. After frustratedly waiting for half an hour, we took another one. We communicated in a mixture of sign language and Yiddish, and I was relieved to part from him when we got back to the hospital. He was returning to Andorra the following day.

Lili called from Bilbao, where they had had to wait for the early, and only, morning plane out. She was disquieted by my depression and promised to return as soon as Ariane was installed with friends and she had attended a concert at Queen Elizabeth Hall, where our son was playing with his Cambridge colleagues.

Monday. The big day on which the dose of Lisuride is to be increased to 2.5mgm. I feel more terrified about it than I had ever anticipated and I think those around me are also behaving strangely. No doctor came, instead, nurses fetched the syringe and indicated that I should place it into the pump myself. I was Off and sitting on the armchair. My head started to buzz and I felt very weak physically. I pulled myself up and went to the toilet. I came back and laid down ready to sleep. The nurse came in and gave me half a Sinemet, which I hadn't expected.

My paranoid feelings know no bounds. I am upset that Obeso hadn't trusted me enough to let me know what he was intending to do, and that neither he nor any other doctor was present to supervise the process. I wanted him to know that I knew, and pressed the bell for the nurse. When she came, I asked her to ask Obeso to take a blood sample, which seemed reasonable if we were to find out what the levels of Lisuride and Sinemet actually were. The time was seven minutes past three. I was frightened in the extreme of dying and that something would crack, or worse still, that I would be left a vegetable.

There was an upsurge of these feelings when the nurse came in to take my temperature and pulse, which was very fast. She said '*no me interesa*' and left. I rang the bell again, and there was a long delay. This time I was told that Dr Obeso was not available but that another doctor was looking for him to ask about the taking of the blood sample. A doctor came in briefly, and I said to tell Obeso that I wasn't a fool, that I knew I'd been given more of the Lisuride than had been agreed.

Still he didn't appear. He was obviously not

coming round, and I felt very angry. What would Dr Parkes think of this treatment?

After a while the worst seemed to be over. I felt more relaxed and walked around. This was reassuring. I was furious that no one had acknowledged that I had been sent on a trip and that I had been left on my own.

As if by miracle, Father Juan appeared in the evening. If I had been a candidate for conversion, this was the moment. Eventually, the overdose showed, and what I felt was intended to be a perfect cure ended up in an excess of facial grimaces and contortions.

Late in the evening, Obeso finally came with a petulant 'What's up?'. I told him I had been through a dreadful experience.

He dealt with it, describing it as a dose variation, and said he wanted to get rid of the 'black areas' (i.e. the Off periods) on the chart and gave me a Sinemet to take. There was no question of his agreeing to my stopping the experiment.

Father Juan, more welcome and kinder than ever, visited me again. 'Just learning his English', he had seen the real crisis, and sensed the danger I felt. He listened to my history, and said he knew very little about psychoanalysis. Nor did he know of Graham Greene whose book I was anxiously reading.

I told Lili on the phone that night that the priest of the Opus Dei had been the only English-speaking human to save me from drug-induced psychosis; she found and brought for him a first edition of Thornton Wilder's *Bridge of San Luis Rey* which is set in the town where he was born.

The following morning, I woke feeling well

enough to get out of bed with an effort. I felt I would like to see how far the Lisuride would take me. I went well till 9 a.m. and then took the delayed pre-breakfast Sinemet. I was supported all along by the knowledge of the *bomba* stuck in my side, as a guiding force, and scolded myself for manufacturing dramas.

The sound of clicking high heels on the marble floor overhead with the expectation, always frustrated, that someone was coming to see me, and the urge to throw myself through the window in my room, kept me walking in the safety of the corridor. To regain some sense of reality and get in touch with the world, I sat down next to a Spaniard who was visiting a relative, but didn't try to make conversation. It seemed that a neurological ward round was taking place, by-passing me. I heard the teaching doctor of the group mutter 'psychologue', and assumed he was referring to me.

I recognized a couple of doctors who had attended me with Dr Obeso and wanted to let them know that I had been On all night until now, and that the drug was effective, but they payed no attention to me. It seemed I was being treated as mad and, unable to defend myself in a language I could not speak, the helplessness surged up in me and I was in a panic. I realized I had to find someone trustworthy to phone Lili in London to come and get me out.

I ran quickly to my room and picked up the phone. I was sure someone was going to prevent me making the call. Lili was fortunately there and I said 'come and get me'. At that moment a woman doctor came to change my syringe and spoke to Lili. I trusted her because she was married, and I presumed, a mother. She told Lili that my agitation was an expectable effect of Lisuride. 'It always does this'. I was relieved and was told that Obeso would come at 3.30 p.m. to explain. He never did.

This, then, was the hallucination I had been sent to test out. When the doctor came to change my syringe, terrified she would put in Largactil, I lay down and looked at the sky to hold on to the world. It seemed as if I was back in a pram once more.

The next day I paced the corridor and had an awareness of a Dali-like floating feeling of a broken brain. That night, at nine o'clock, Lili arrived by taxi from Bilbao and I felt safer with someone on my side. She did not leave me again, sleeping in the bed chair which at last came into its own.

She came too late to catch Obeso, but her call from London insisting on a lowering of the dosage was respected next morning.

We waited all next day for Obeso, who was in the building, but wouldn't come. He arrived late in the evening, and said he had talked to the drug company in Berlin who would ensure I would get supplies in London. He said that what had happened to me was due to my isolation away from home and not knowing Spanish, rather than the failure of his team. He seemed to have washed his hands of me and my paranoia which, he simply couldn't and didn't handle. Used as I was to the discipline of training and working in a teaching hospital in England, I felt there was something missing in this establishment. A psychiatrist should have been on hand to monitor the side effects and their relation to dose.

As we approached the last days of my adventure (I was to be discharged at the end of the week), I had the strangest experience of all. Lili and I were whiling away the time outside my room, when group after group of doctors passed by on their way to or from their rounds. Then Dr Obeso appeared, accompanied by a man in a grey business suit. Seeing me, he made a detour towards me and pointing to me, said to the man beside him: 'You know Dr Todes?' I couldn't believe my eyes. It was Dr Stern. Even Lili was shocked, so unlikely a situation did we find ourselves in.

I was quite sure, of course, that he had been summoned to certify me and discount me as a witness against Lisuride, and their team experimenting with it. We all went into my room and Stern chatted amiably with me and I commented angrily on Dr Obeso's liking for trick playing. I said it would have been courteous to warn me of my own doctor's arrival in Spain. I challenged him on his visit. Why had he come? He said the purpose of his visit was to see the Lisuride programme which he intended to try out in his unit in eight months' time.

My obviously distressed state and my feverish look made him uncomfortable; so, as quickly as protocol permitted, after some small talk, he turned to the door and edged out of the room and, giving my hand a shake, said he was sorry I was having such a rough time.

Lili, aghast, ran down the corridor after him. She said to him how sick I was and how frightened we both felt. His response, as he turned and proceeded down the corridor, was compassionate, 'Poor man!' She then stopped Obeso and asked if I would recover. Barely raising his eyes from his clip-board, he said, 'I hope so'. This was no reassurance.

Neither of us knew what to do to get out from there safely and speedily. Safely, because Lili rightly worried about the effects of suddenly stopping a drug of this order, and also because I was not really well enough to travel.

We had one last meeting with Obeso, who wrote prescriptions and a shopping list for the pump, syringes, iodine, plaster and the cotton pocket to hold it all. He also suggested a certificate for customs. After the experience I had been through, we were not likely to ever use the drug again in that particular form, but wanted to maintain the pretence. We queued up in the administrative office for the bill.

We left the hospital before dawn, bolting from the oppression of my experience. My last definitive action had been to rip off the plaster band that cradled the pump, and finally to take out the needle from my abdomen. We crept, like felons, out of the goods lift with our bags, to a waiting taxi. It took us through the cool sunrise to Bilbao, passing the flat scrubland and wind-swept plains of Navarra tinged in pink. The city, dank and polluted even at dawn, with its obsolete scarred docks and its rusting iron hulls was evocative of the 1930s with shades of Brecht and Weil with Lotte Lenya singing the Bilbao song in the musical *Happy End*.

So anxious had we been to make our escape from the hospital that we arrived before the small airport had opened its doors to passengers, and watched the staff preparing for their day, putting on their uniforms and opening the ticket check-ins. The wooden expressions of the customs and emigration officials were threatening; for me, it was a continuation of the paranoid world I had been submerged in; I felt I was expected to make a run for it to safety and freedom across a mythological border.

Instead, we merely boarded the plane for a routine two-hour flight to Gatwick. The gentle air hostess on board reassured me. I was feeling physically very ill and fragile. I still felt wrapped in the confinement of my ward. I certainly didn't feel secure until I was back within the safety of my home, and reunited with my children.

The cache of medical equipment we had purchased from the pharmacist next to the hospital remains untouched on the bottom shelf of the medicine cupboard gathering dust, a totem of the bad days gone by. Nobody quite dares throw them away.

After a couple of days in bed blowing off the remaining Lisuride in my system, I returned on Monday to report to Dr Parkes for a debriefing. Stroking his left eyebrow with the knuckle of his little finger, he said it was as he had expected. He confirmed that he had had similar experiences with patients on Lisuride in the way of psychotic side effects. I never quite understood why with this knowledge he had underwritten my trip to Pamplona. But I was a persuasive witness in favour of his argument with his chief (David Marsden) not to persist with the experiment. We agreed that a psychiatrist should be included in the team during attempts to stabilize patients on Lisuride. I had a letter in *The Lancet* to that effect, and there was general agreement in the correspondence that followed.

Dr Suchy, the physician involved with the marketing of Lisuride, flew over from Berlin for lunch at our house to hear all about the experience and was sympathetic. Her firm, Schering, agreed to meet the expenses of my hospitalization in Pamplona.

CHAPTER 11

Three Wise Men

I returned to London to find a brief but stinging letter awaiting me from my colleagues at the Paddington Centre. They had been misinformed by the administration that I was returning to work after three weeks of sick leave instead of the six months' leave I had applied for before going to Pamplona.

The letter referred to this confusion, and asked *me* to put it right. Using the error as a pretext, they renewed their plea to resign my post on the grounds of ill-health, with a scarcely hooded threat, once again invoking the Three Wise Men procedure. In real terms, it represented a court martial. It was a humiliating threat and an unjustified one. I felt extremely incensed by this device to attack my competence as a means of ridding themselves of me. It spoilt the many years of dedicated and appreciated work that I had contributed to the community. I felt I knew my limitations as well as my capabilities and was hopeful that, with the benefit of treatment for a continuity of response to the drug, I could improve and maintain those capabilities enough to continue in my job. In the event I stayed away for six months, on the recommendation of Dr Parkes, to recoup the strength lost as a result of the Lisuride trial.

The NHS unit manager came to my home in early August. We discussed the fact that no medical objection had been tabled by the district physician responsible for staff health, and the unit manager agreed that it was not my Parkinson's disease as much as the hostile environment that had developed against me at the clinic. He discussed the possibility of finding alternative sessions in the district.

I had consulted the district manager herself before my departure for Spain and asked her for sessions elsewhere. She said that this resiting would prove to be no problem.

On 10 August I steeled myself to a return to the clinic. I found a huge bouquet of roses on my desk from my wife with the legend: 'When the going gets tough, the tough get going'. Next to it was a little scrawled note from one unsubstantial clinic psychologist, pleading that for the survival of the clinic and for my own good, I should reconsider my return. Upstairs in the bleak room where the meeting was held, I received a colder welcome still. I was expecting to join the unit manager and the other doctors to help sort out how to overcome the difficulties of the clinic, which were approaching a climax.

Instead, I was stunned to learn that the unit manager, who greeted me, had just put down the phone to summon to the meeting the district physician responsible for staff health. I had seen him a year earlier, in a confidential interview, and then he had found no grounds for my not resuming my work. His presence would seem to have made a nonsense out of the confidentiality, which is so dear to the medical profession. It seems obvious, now, that this was a compromise on behalf of my colleagues, who wanted direct action to remove me. When the district physician came, he recommended that I return on trial for two months, and that my work should be monitored by a colleague. A further attempt to highlight my deficiencies was made when they insisted on my chairing the weekly children's department meeting. Chairing meetings was never my strong point, even without the PD. It was another ill-conceived ploy to undermine my confidence. I went home in a rage and wrote a letter to the unit manager expressing my dismay at the devious and deplorable treatment I had received and adding:

> I should like to say that my PD is being supervised by an eminent neurologist specialist in PD, whom I see regularly and who has encouraged me and agreed to my resumption of my work after the setback I had experienced as a result of the trial. You should know that if he felt the work too heavy, I would be the first to hand in my resignation.
>
> As to the monitoring of my work, I would refer to my records and notes on the patients under my care after fourteen years of my disability and suggest that if there are any indications from that for monitoring, to please point this out, and let's put an end to the innuendos once and for all. Could I then not be allowed to do my work free from pressure and have the trust that I enjoyed before?

I added that I confessed to having delegated the chair of the department to a more adept person some years ago, not at the best of times possessing a talent for committees.

In this intolerable atmosphere I resumed my work, doing four sessions instead of six to accommodate the other consultant and coping with my share of the administrative work.

My letter, of which the first copy was 'lost', I discovered later, was interpreted as showing my 'inability to grasp issues and to come to conclusions when presented with certain facts'.

Meantime, the clinic remained under threat of closure, with redundancies so long threatened now becoming a reality. The district manager never responded to either phone calls or recorded delivery letters. I confined myself to my work with patients, the staff and school doctors that I supervised. Nobody spoke to me and in this isolation, the teamwork and clinic activities ceased to be enjoyable.

The pressures put on me by the administration together with the conduct of my colleagues succeeded. I was left with no alternative. My advisers at the BMA negotiated the retirement, forgetting that I was now on four sessions rather than the six I had done for nearly twenty years. As the pension was based on the best years' earnings in the last three years, I failed to get my full entitlement. This fact also reduced my redundancy pay by a third. After a hefty exchange of correspondence and meetings involving district politics which included reports from colleagues unknown to me and, therefore, against which I could not defend myself, I left the clinic in the New Year of 1987.

CHAPTER 12

Vienna Again

While I was struggling to keep my job, in face of my colleagues' attempt to scuttle me, my fight on the Parkinson's disease front continued. I knew I could respond better to the events by obtaining continuity from my medication, and thus become less vulnerable to attack.

I began to relax and recover my strength. By my own efforts and with the encouragement of my family, my work with patients and in my private practice went well.

In 1986 we arranged a holiday in Vienna to coincide with our children attending master classes given annually by a Russian violin teacher at the Konservatorium.

Knowing that we were going to be in Vienna, it seemed a good idea to inquire about neurological research in Austria. The prompting came from a *Jewish Chronicle* article, which had a small column claiming that a professor of pharmacology had found a cure for Parkinson's disease. I recognized the name of Prof. Youdim. I had visited him at the Haifa Technikon in Israel some years earlier and I phoned him. He shrugged off the report, saying that the facts were completely misrepresented, but mentioned that he was to attend a conference in Vienna at the end of September where Prof. Walter Birkmayer would be presenting his work involving the enzyme Tyrosine hydroxylase. An enzyme is a chemical that facilitates a reaction between chemicals without being changed itself. By chemically suppressing this enzyme more dopamine becomes available to the brain.

When asked on the telephone, Prof. Youdim thought that this involved injections with a special form of iron. Youdim had collaborated with Birkmayer in the research on Deprenyl and had high regard for his hunches, which, he said, usually turned out to be correct. This seemed a good endorsement from an experienced and serious worker in the field, and despite my reluctance to start another trial, I thought I would investigate the possibilities.

So once again, and this time without apprehension, the three-ring circus of myself, my wife and Ariane set off in high spirits by ferry to Ostend and there entrained into the sleeper to Cologne. After the rather dull landscapes of Belgium, the journey along the Rhine was magical. The turreted castles and sloping vineyards of the great river unwound alongside our carriage and people in pleasure boats waved in the direction of our train. We stopped off in the Bavarian town of Bamberg, where my wife was born. I had had a mental picture of it from her nostalgic description of significant places in her life, particularly the thirteenth-century cathedral. The cathedral overlooks the small town from one of its seven hills; a sculpture of the Bamberg Rider on horseback dominates the nave, and there is a carved stone figure of a blindfolded woman with a staff called 'Synagogue', or blind justice. Next to the cathedral is the palace of the prince bishops of Bavaria and there are large formal gardens filled with the scent of thousands of roses. Two arms of a river enclose the baroque part of Bamberg below. The sound of running water is everywhere.

The house, on the tree-lined avenue where she was born and lived until she and her family had to escape from the Nazis, had been transformed into a printing house. We had contact with a former playmate who had prospered in the war, but for the rest, I regarded it as a museum city of great beauty, but with a stained heart.

We spent four days in Bamberg, my wife rediscovering memories from her childhood, while I indulged myself in a diet of würst, bier and krapfen (pancakes) at the attractive beer halls and eating houses.

And so to Vienna, where we met up with my son Rafael, who already had begun his violin course and was pleased to guide us around central areas of the Ring and the good, inexpensive restaurants he had sniffed out. The city had been developed in the 1840s, like Haussmann's Paris, in the shape of a circle, making crowd control easier in any revolution, when the guns could be pointed and rapidly shifted to different radials of the circle.

We stayed at a pension a few minutes away from the opera house, the Hofburg and the cathedral. At night, the sound of the carriages carrying tourists on the narrow cobbled street below reverberated against the buildings and kept us awake. I was glad to be back, after my traumatic experience of 1971.

Change was not very noticeable in the way of new buildings, the old façades remaining as solid reminders of the vanished Austro-Hungarian imperial tradition. We enjoyed evenings at the Volksoper, and visited the home of

Sigmund Freud at 19 Berggasse, now established as a museum.

We phoned Prof. Birkmayer at the state-run clinic, the Evangelisches Krankenhaus, where he consulted and made an appointment with his secretary. The clinic, overlooking the canal, a tramride away from the pension and not far from the Freud house in the Berggasse, had been built between the wars and looked a little dilapidated. The terrazzo floor in the entrance, which acted as a waiting room, looked chipped and the paint was peeling. We were invited to join the other couples lining this entrance area by a nurse, and learned from them how revered the professor was.

He has a passion for medicine and a reputation for being a miracle worker. To him all patients are equally important; numbered among them, Mao and Franco; while Brezhnev's physician was reported to have consulted Birkmayer. At seventy-six, his slight and agile figure is familiar on the ski slopes most winter weekends, and the tennis courts and the ballroom the rest of the year. His television appearances make him a well-known personality to all Viennese, as we discovered.

When he arrived, there was a flutter of hand kissing and warm greetings directed in friendly inquiry to waiting patients as though they were old acquaintances. Prof. Birkmayer is of medium height, athletic and slim, his tanned bald head surrounded by a wispish line of white hair.

He went briefly into his consulting room, and emerged presently in a white theatre gown. 'Come in, my dear colleague', he said, welcoming us with an outstretched hand and ushering us inside. His desk was in the middle of a room divided into four cubicles by curtained partitions, and he invited me to sit down next to him. In response to his query, I described my medical history and my current drug dosages, which he noted down. He knew my neurologists well from international conferences where he met regularly with them. Indeed, he had recently ceded the editorship of an international journal to David Parkes who, he added with amusement, had just rejected a paper he had submitted. Dr Parkes said later in London, when I reported back, that Birkmayer was having a little joke.

Then, in a serious vein, he described his new medication which was given intravenously. He didn't clarify too much, scribbling his theory on a scrap of paper in his flamboyant style, telling me that he would be presenting a paper on this treatment in Vienna in October, and that he had a paper on it accepted for publication in an American journal. The treatment used a tri-valent iron (instead of the usual di-valent) to act on Tyrosine hydroxylase. This was achieved through the use of oxyferriscorbone, a French preparation used in France for treatment of severe anaemia. He said he didn't yet have supplies to pursue all his experiments and suggested I phone him in the middle of September to find out whether they had arrived.

I phoned him some weeks later from London and he said he now had some supplies and invited me to come to Vienna for a series of treatments. I felt that this gentle and vivacious Viennese professor, of whom three top neurologists said he had never been wrong, would provide a last-ditch rescue from my forced retirement. Indeed, he had been involved in Carbidopa, Deprenyl, as well as in pioneering work with L-dopa.

Once again, armed with my On/Off charts for the professor's guidance, and with guarded hopes and presents, we were on our way to Vienna. This time we flew. We had booked, at the suggestion of the professor's nurse, at the Hotel Mozart, near to the clinic and opposite one of the railway stations. It was large and seedy, a place for day-trippers from across the border in Hungary, who arrived with plastic bags containing consumer goods and filled the lounges and available space with dense cigarette smoke and excited talk.

We stayed only one night in the broken-down room with the leak from a water pipe creeping towards our bed. Where to go? We remembered a man with whom we had shared a taxi from the airport being deposited at a Hotel Strudelhof not far away. We walked there and to our delight found a modern hotel, designed for OPEC diplomats, nestling in the grounds of the palace owned by Count Strudelhof. For the next eight glorious autumn days, we found perfect peace and contentment in the quiet room and green surroundings, not far from the little tram that plied the Ring, and near enough to the professor's ministering.

We had agreed that as an outpatient, I would attend his clinic at ten o'clock each morning. On most mornings, the nurse was busily applying herself between three beds. She had great experience in intravenous work and went about it with effective gusto. I mounted the bed by means of a two-step cream painted wooden block. She then twisted a rubber tourniquet round my arm and inserted an inverted bottle, with its needle attached, into my vein over the elbow. She never had difficulty in finding a vein, and showed skill and speed that was masterly. The professor told us she was a former ice-skating champion; I should suspect that she would excel equally well at darts. As the amber-coloured solution entered my vein I had a great feeling of being well and relaxed, and felt myself getting pinker in the face. The rest of the day, we were left to our own devices. After a week's treatment with the iron, my condition was not improved. If anything, it had deteriorated. I ascribed this to my taking myself off the Pergolide and Deprenyl in order to see what response there would be to the injected material. I shuffled beside my wife through the enchanting streets and monuments of Vienna. Each evening, we presented ourselves at the opera box office where the subscribers, who were unable to attend, sold their prized tickets. These tickets were for seats not always with full vision of the stage. But the sound came round wonderfully and the occasion was always memorable, and somehow, my drug always worked. In the interval the promenade of the Viennese in their showy, sparkling gowns were a tribute, if not to haute coûture, to individuality of expression and a childlike desire to show off.

They raised the dose of iron after the second day. The plan was to get further supplies from France where it was on sale from most pharmacies. Birkmayer suggested that I contact Dr Stern who might supervise the continuation of the infusions for four weeks after my return.

I didn't feel the support between doses which I relied on from the agonist drug, Pergolide. On the penultimate day, I decided that since no clear picture emerged from the iron alone, I would resume taking the agonist. It was when I was with the professor that I had a reaction to my agonist and turned pale. He sat me down and waited reassuringly, taking my pulse. Soon I was better, but it taught me to treat this useful but tricky medication with respect.

Apart from this episode, I had enough good feeling about the iron to continue with it back home. Prof. Birkmayer could give me one week's supply of the injectable material. In London, I met with Dr Stern and he was willing for the experiment to continue, offering facilities and manpower at the Middlesex Hospital. He added a delightful vignette about the venerable professor: when made honorary president of the International Society for Neurology, Birkmayer thanked the members and said he would only agree to take it for a limited period of twenty-five years.

A registrar at the Middlesex Hospital injected the iron three times a week. When the professor's supply ran out, knowing it was freely available for anaemics in France, Lili went on a day-trip to Boulogne by ferry and bought twenty packets of the iron. The astonished pharmacist had clearly never heard of the application of this inexpensive help, which was usually given to someone vomiting blood, now being used in the treatment of Parkinson's disease.

When a medical colleague heard about the quantities of iron involved, he alerted me to the risk of subjecting myself to an overload of iron with the hazard of damage to the tissues involved. An appointment was arranged for a consultation with Dr Huehns, a haematologist. Huehns took blood to ascertain levels of iron and recommended that I stop the infusions, fearing iron overload and damage to the liver and kidneys. This would be a poor trade-off against the limited and indeed questionable benefits of the iron treatment. Once again my enthusiasm for benefit had led me into hazardous treatment, whose proponents blinded me to its real value and dangerous side effects.

CHAPTER 13

Transplant

From the early days of treatment with drugs, I felt that the daily doses of chemical replacement were too untargeted and diffuse; the On-Off effects and the dyskinesia were ultimately soul-destroying, and making life increasingly circumscribed. I had to face the fact that the striatal cells would continue to degenerate and that the final neurotransmitter bridge was flimsy, making me completely dependent on drugs for the connection.

If, in some perverse and unpredictable way, the drug failed to shunt in on time, whether delayed by gastric irritability, a heavy meal, enzyme competition for transportation to the brain or factor x, I was stranded and only barely mobile. How often did I find myself in my dinner suit, all primed for a party, sitting in the car or driving about outside, waiting for the drug to come through. Life with Parkinson's disease was a continual inner personal battle of trying to gain greater stability on drugs.

The precarious balance between being Off and being On, and moving into dyskinesia (grimaces) was very difficult to achieve. The expected duration of benefit from a morning dose is about two hours. After that the follow-up needs to be taken after an hour and so forth.

The demands of daily work in my practice were invaluable; work and its requirements were often the best motivators. It is still a mystery how the ring of the front door bell summons up unsuspected reserves of neurotransmitter. The pressure to remain On led to overdosing, and the dyskinesia that followed was far more unpleasant than being Off. Biological processes that occurred with daily regulatory (circadian rhythms) seemed to be at work, so that lower and more frequent doses were required in the morning, and a rest needed in the afternoon if one hoped to be active in the evening.

The personal outer battle to keep up, left me having to peddle twice as fast in order to stay on the same spot, and yet the nature of the illness was such that a good proportion of the time one could barely peddle adequately.

Without the motivation of attending the clinic daily and facing a variety of problem-solving situations and activities with a team, I found my available physical and mental energy increasingly limited. I directed more attention and strength into hopes for the future and means of realizing them.

Perhaps one of the few advantages of the fully developed condition was that I now seemed to be less troubled by sleepiness. However, medication taken late at night produced a driven effect of excitation and dyskinesia and troubled my rest. Mobility in bed was much less of a problem since a friend gave me an electric bed which jacked me up from a horizontal to a sitting position and, combined with an overhead monkeyhold, helped me in turning from side to side and getting out of bed. I feel I know every corner of my bed and how to get to it.

At this stage of the illness, I felt it useful to separate the different modes of feeling and thinking associated with the On-Off:

The first response to the drug in the morning, approximately half an hour after intake, is one of well-being and energy. I feel integrated and in touch with past experience and also oriented towards the future and capable of leading an active and competitive life. The follow-up pills already hint at increasing tension and grimacing. The imagination rigidifies and there is a hint of anxiety and depression; although I am On and appear to be normal, I feel rather tense.

With the wearing off of the drug's benefits, reactive backlash produces momentary but profoundly negative feelings. When these pass, or when they have not appeared, I experience fatigue and dependence – infantile feelings related to immobility. It is as if one's psychological skin bristles with being restricted, like when one was a little child.

At best, in this state, there is no further drop in the level of neurotransmitters, and some hope emerges. Intellect dominates as mobility diminishes, because problems solved in the head are not readily translated into action. Although frustrating, this helplessness can be accepted now, in a way which wouldn't have been possible in the early stages of the illness. It would appear that the chemistry of protest, the four 'f's, has been neutralized and a passionless acquiesence predominates.

Dementia, which I had anticipated with terror, has not emerged. What has become clear, is a generalized passivity with the appearance of physical debility. This is very different from feeble-mindedness and true dementia.

With the positive reaction to the drug, connection to mobility is made and with it comes the reassurance that I am once more part of the family of man, rather than a mere dodo. The soul has been chemically restored, reminding me that life without motion and emotion is tantamount to living death. However, even with the best skill, time-keeping and regularity, there remained side effects and an unpredictability to this treatment that made me look in another direction.

The obvious solution seemed to me to be to replace the actual degenerating striatal cells of the corpus striatum which were failing to produce the neurotransmitter, dopamine. The replacement would come from aborted foetal brain cells or from synthetically developed material. The idea of transplanting organs, or, at a lower level of differentiation, specialized tissue cells, lay in the domain of the fantasists and science fiction writers. Kidney transplants had already taken place but they had not captured the public's interest in a major way. Then Christian Barnard and his team startled the world by performing an operation in which the heart of a newly dead patient was implanted in a nearly dead one. There were problems of rejection by the body's immune system to overcome, but, by the late 1970s, many units around the world were performing organ transplants. At a cellular level, babies were being produced after fertilization in test tubes by Steptoe and Edwards.

It was at this time that I read in a newspaper about a publication by Prof. Mark Perlow on work he had done on rats at St Elizabeth Hospital in Washington, DC. They were rendered Parkinsonian on one side and implanted with embryonic tissue. The paper he published showed that the result of the work on rats was apparently gratifying. No rejection had taken place after eight months and the graft took and secreted dopamine and possibly other substances, yet to be identified. I wrote to Dr Perlow and offered myself as a willing, and I thought useful, subject for human trials when he was ready to do them.

To my disappointment, no reply came from Washington. I then wrote to Dr Barnard, thinking that, with his high profile and prestige, he would get things moving:

Dear Prof. Barnard:

I write to you with the foreknowledge of your expressed interest in the idea of brain tissue transplants and particularly your pre-eminence and pioneering work in the field of transplants.

I am a 48-year-old child psychiatrist, father of three, and gradually being worn down by a predominantly left-sided Parkinson's disease. It occurred to me that if ever a condition called for a transplant, this one does – after all, the area has been well explored by neurosurgeons doing various pallidal and thalamic sections, so this would not present insuperable problems. The defective tissue is circumscribed neuro-secretory rather than neuro-conducting, possibly making success more likely and less complicated. Failure, if well carried out, should not leave the structure worse.

I enclosed a reprint of Perlow's paper, and said that while he might consider himself to be outside the neurosurgical field, his courage and experience with all the ramifications of such research, would make him an ideal coordinator of such an operation.

I added my conviction that the procedure would eventually be done and for myself, the sooner the better.

There was no response from Prof. Barnard either.

Through the good offices of a patient of mine I was put in touch with Irving Cooper. He had pioneered the thalamotomy* operation to relieve PD tremor by stereotactic** brain surgery. This form of treatment had been selectively used with varying degrees of success before the advent of L-dopa, but was abandoned in favour of the newly discovered drug.

Dr Cooper was still practising in the United States and he, in turn, put me in touch with Prof. Watkins at the London Hospital who relayed to me his feelings that 'we have not yet reached the point where we would be prepared to perform the procedure'. He did an assessment of my condition and ordered IQ tests to be done so as to have them for comparisons, should surgery be contemplated later.

The next hint of excitement came in 1981 when it was announced, from the Karolinska Institute in Stockholm, that an implant into the brain using the patient's own adrenal medullary material*** (autograft) for their dopamine-producing cells, was about to be attempted. The basic tissue preparation had been done at Lund University in Sweden by Anders Bjorkland, and the surgeon involved was Prof. Backlund. The surgery was done stereotactically, that is, using special X-rays of the skull, with the patient harnessed to a metallic frame so as to pinpoint the site for the

---

* Creating a lesion (cut) in the dorso-medial nucleus of the thalamus using stereotactic devices.

** Use of a stainless steel frame screwed into the bony cranium to assess by stereo X-rays any exact point in the brain.

*** The adrenal medulla is the central part of the adrenal gland which sits on the kidney and contains dopamine-producing cells which have been transplanted into the brain in PD. The advantage is that rejection problems are avoided but fatalities have occurred frequently.

operation, in all dimensions. The tissue, taken surgically from the patient, from an area above the kidney was placed in the region of the striatum, alongside the caudate nucleus and stapled to it.

The operation was performed in Stockholm, Sweden, on the first of three selected patients, at the end of March, 1981. The patient did not show any sign of improvement, and although the rigidity was reduced at first, he soon had to return to the same dose of medication as before surgery. However, this pioneering work of grafting living cells into a damaged brain evoked great excitement because no rejection had taken place. I began to initiate moves to be among the selected patients chosen for the procedure in the future.

I corresponded with Prof. Backlund. One day, I received a telephone call from a TV director, Alan Patient, telling me that Prof. Backlund had agreed to his operation being filmed for BBC TV when the next adrenal autograft would take place at the Karolinska Institute (Patient had already had a look around the Institute and was impressed). Over an alcoholic luncheon at home, involving all the family for the purpose of the film, we all became very excited about the prospect for myself, the BBC, the professor and all sufferers of Parkinson's disease. The possibility of failure seemed remote.

In the event, the protocol to be followed in the experiment of the remaining two operations with carefully monitored patients, fared no better and no film was made. But I did meet Prof. Backlund in Bergen, where he had now accepted the chair of neurosurgery, and where my family and I spent a summer holiday.

He rates high on my list of people I have come across in my search for help with my Parkinson's disease. He received us at Haukeland Hospital in his high-tech, beautifully appointed department, at short notice and with great warmth and courtesy. He took us to his lecture theatre and showed a film of the operation he and his team had done, explaining it step by step. He regretted that his results showed no noticeable improvements but felt it was a vital link in the chain to ultimate success. He was unwilling, on religious grounds, to experiment with human foetuses, but did think that the nerve growth factor plus cloned cells might be the preferred method. I felt that his consummate skill and his integrity, as evidenced in his operation, kept him on a straight line of research in which some day he is bound to succeed. In his quiet, understated way, he supports one with tremendous strength and inspires confidence. He thought, seeing me in an On state, that I was too fit to experiment on with untried and unknown methods. Certainly, from his demonstration and commentary, both my wife and I received some underlying confidence in this type of procedure.

Suddenly, the transplant scene was enlivened by the results of a series of adrenal medullary autografts done by Madrazzo in Mexico City. The press reports were overwhelmingly dramatic and seductive. 'Parkinson's Disease Cured', screamed the headlines, and wealthy friends offered to send me post-haste to Mexico City. The patient who was 'cured' was now able to play football with his son, which evidently he was unable to do before. The reputable New England *Journal of Medicine* reported favourably on Madrazzo's work – but two of his patients did infact die following the operation.

This operation was soon replicated all over the United States while Madrazzo carried out a foetal cell transplant, for which he also claimed success. The foetal cell transplant was banned in the United States, by President Reagan himself, in any institution funded federally, pending an inquiry which was to report at the end of the year. The ban remains under President Bush, but privately funded experiments are taking place at Yale and in Colorado. This coincided with the first British transplant on Betty Knight in March 1988.

The transplant had been my main hope over a ten-year period, and once there was no success from the Scandinavian effort, I began agitating for it in London. Dr Andrew Lees was interested in transplants. I had been treated by him when he was senior registrar to Dr Stern at UCH at the beginning of the Pergolide experiment, and I had seen him regularly for follow-ups. Then I collaborated with him on the production of a paper on personality as a factor in PD. His work on transplantation was carried out with Mr David Thomas, neurosurgeon at Queen's Square, with whom I discussed the transplant. He was clearly in no hurry to get into action. I think his view was that it would take five to ten years before any significant development would occur. Their work was being done on marmosets. Steven Dunnett at Cambridge was involved in research on the histological side, that is, tissue culture.

One problem in striatal transplants was to do with possible tissue rejection by the receiver's immune system, although it was thought that the brain tissue would have privileged status as far as rejection was concerned. There was some fear, too, about the growth of foetal cells becoming rampant and how to stop this. Further unease was to do with the use of foetal material; this might run counter to the anti-abortion lobby, which at the time was endeavouring to have abortion after sixteen weeks outlawed by parliament. As animal experiment pointed to the use of foetal cells of ten weeks and under, this would not pose a problem in itself. Nevertheless, the climate in parliament and the press reflected nervousness over the use of aborted material.

Meanwhile, David Marsden, who had been appointed to the chair at Queens' Square, made a link with Swedish workers at Lund and Stockholm. The British contribution to the joint work was access to the PET scan, an expensive and unique apparatus that can determine the course of development of any transplant by means of radioactive cell markers. It was the proud possession of the Hammersmith Hospital in West London. The London group were slowly accumulating animal data in preparation for an operation to be done after the Swedes had reported the results of their transplant operations, one year on.

Their leisurely approach must have been severely jolted by the banner headlines on 18 April, 1988, announcing a cure for Parkinson's disease. Inside, the picture and story of Betty Knight, who had been chairbound and moribund before being rescued by Professor Hitchcock, who was known to be a world authority on the stereotactic approach to brain surgery. His special interest in Parkinson's disease came as a surprise. It dated from five years back when Dr Chris Clough, neurological registrar at the East Midland unit, was disappointed by the helplessness of some chronic Parkinson's patients. They did a pilot animal study, and waited for a year or two for the ethical committee of the hospital to agree to a series of trials to be done using foetal cells. Betty Knight was the first beneficiary of this venture.

My excitement was unbounded when I read that what I had pursued around the world was now available a short distance from home, in Birmingham. I immediately phoned my friend John Coop, a fellow Parkinsonian. He agreed that someone heroic enough to have attempted such a breakthrough needed support. We both sent off telegrams.

In my congratulatory message, I asked to be considered as a candidate for a graft. I was astonished to receive an answer by return, expressing appreciation at my message. In a follow-up letter, Prof. Hitchcock invited me to make an appointment for assessment.

Wide coverage of the Birmingham operation had set in motion another wave of discussion and condemnation of the use of foetal tissue. I wrote a letter to my MP alerting him to the breakthrough to overcome Parkinson's disease by surgical means and the threat by the anti-abortion lobby at this early stage of the experimental work. I strongly defined to him my personal view on the ethics involved and requested it should be made very clear in debate in the House that:

1. The cells are taken from dead foetuses.
2. The tissue involved is equivalent to an organ transplant, or even, at a more acceptable level, a blood transfusion (this still remains unacceptable to a small minority of people).
3. Abortions are not infrequent in the natural course of events, and the striatal cells of these may eventually be used at this stage, rather than hazarding fundamental experiment with possibly sick cells.
4. Prof. Hitchcock has used cells from an elective abortion.
5. Under no circumstances would a decision about abortion be influenced by the needs of a patient for transplant.
6. As in heart transplants, separate teams are involved in the decision-making.
7. The use of foetal material, which would generally be headed for the incinerator, should be kept very separate from the issue of abortion.

I drew his attention to the fact that this simple, elegant surgery, pioneered in Sweden, if successful, would eliminate vast costs of treatment of chronic, long-term illnesses for the many sufferers. I cited my own experience of the unreliability of drugs forcing my premature retirement at fifty-five. I pleaded that hysteria and the omnipresent spectre of Frankenstein should not hamper an operation which might reduce the heavy burden of cost on the medical facilities, and add useful working years to the careers of young Parkinsonians.

His reply was swift and unequivocal; he would give his complete support 'along the lines' I indicated.

CHAPTER 14

Doubts and Delays

I rang up Prof. Hitchcock's secretary, Veronica Taylor, and made an appointment for Wednesday, 18 May, at the East Midland Centre for Neurosurgery and Neurology at Smethwick.

It came as a surprise that the appointment was made so readily, given the massive interest resulting from the television coverage. I was exhilarated. Soon, however, depression and doubts took over.

There was to be an International Congress on Parkinson's disease in Jerusalem that summer, at which the latest developments in the field would be on show. I knew from an

American neurologist about a new internal delivery system for L-dopa which, by bringing a loop of the small bowel onto the surface of the abdomen for insertion of the drug, would, it was hoped, bypass the liver circulation and do away with the oscillations. No doubt other advances would be presented by researchers. I spoke to Prof. Backlund by telephone and he said he knew from the grapevine that the two foetal implants in the joint Swedish-London study had not shown any improvement in the patients.

Despite these promises and considerations, I decided to attend the appointment in Birmingham, rationalizing it as a fact-finding interview with options to undergo the operation, should it be offered, after the results of the first three trials had shown something positive.

On the 9.40 a.m. commuter train from Euston nerves really overtook my wife. We agreed between ourselves that I would make no commitment until we had met and spent time with at least one of the subjects, and that, in any case, we would wait and see the results.

We arrived in Birmingham with the other commuters after a speedy journey of one hour and forty minutes. With the milling crowds, we spent some time running up and down the litter-strewn stairs before we found the platform for the local train. The remainder of the way took in tough areas, scrap-metal depots, corrugated roofs of small workshops and graffiti sprayed over every surface, just like in London. It was as if a sort of superman on wings, with a spray gun, had worked his way from empty space to empty space till there was none left.

We crossed the rickety wooden footbridge at Smethwick, and from the station we had a steep twenty minutes' uphill walk through streets lined with gaudily painted rows of houses. I reflected that if all went well, we'd be seeing a lot of these houses and these streets in the months to come.

It was midday and the air was bracing. Shades of

Pamplona! Eventually after skirting a large park (of which there are many in the suburbs of Birmingham), we came upon the hospital.

Approached from the main road, the sprawling red-brick Victorian building is set back in a large old orchard. Its isolated position, surrounded by a tall brick wall, overgrown with ivy, and adjacent to a cemetery, told of its history as a fever hospital. Under the leaden sky, it was a gloomy reception.

In the more modern annexe to the main building, we had a cheerier welcome from the neurologist, Dr Clough, who was waiting for us in the outpatients' department. He took us into a suite of consulting rooms the minute we arrived. Young, slender and engaging, he opened a pink folder and began writing the expanding history of my Parkinson's disease.

He was intrigued and fascinated. He was also very frank about the work they were doing. It was proving exciting, but inconclusive, he said. He would not pretend otherwise. No result could be guaranteed, and there were the obvious risks involved in a brain operation – paralysis, bleeding and infection. It was too early to know what the long-term, and indeed the short-term, results from the two patients would show. That very day the team were performing the operation on a third patient.

We discussed the latest developments in the treatment of Parkinson's disease, the personalities involved and their approaches to research and its application. He said there were three possible outcomes: death, no change in the condition, or, improvement. The gamble was on the latter two. He then proceeded to a physical examination and, adjusting his large-framed turquoise spectacles, told my wife that I was remarkably fit, before leaving to fetch his chief. Suddenly, with the rush of air that surrounds VIPs, the professor swept into the room, followed by his secretary.

His hand outstretched, he pre-empted my greeting by saying, 'Your telegram was the only one I replied to'.

I recognized him instantly from his television appearances. The same confidence in the face of questioning, the tilt of the head crowned by a thick mane of greying black hair, and a great charm in giving his response. He was of medium height, slim in build, and, under the brisk manner, there was a worn look around his eyes. He impressed me as open and direct.

He had been briefed by the neurologist. I was an ideal candidate; under sixty-five, disease not too bad, highly motivated and cooperative, an excellent subject for research. He said he had had eight hundred inquiries since Betty Knight's case came to the public's attention.

I asked him many questions which he answered, often saying quite frankly that he did not know. He said he had two reservations about taking me on: one was that, from a glance at my records, he could see that I 'fiddle with my drugs'; the second, that I lived too far away, which would make difficulties for the follow-up research to which I would have to submit. He warned me that the post-operative tests would include periodical lumbar punctures, to obtain samples of cerebro-spinal fluid, as this was the only accessible way to determine the dopamine level in the brain apart from a PET scan. At that time they had no access to a scanner which, by the use of radioactive fluorodopa, can measure the actual secretory capacity of the striatal cells and use the information as a comparison before and after implant. I was being wooed, all this time, with the shared knowledge, and challenged with the lack of it. The disarming response to my inquiries being, more often than not, 'we don't know'.

I told him I wondered what happens to foetal graft cells if they multiply without control, or have unknown or unchartered properties. He dismissed it as mythology and said that their problem was not too many but too few cells; if an excess of cells should cause a tumour, they were experienced enough to operate. We spoke about Prof. Backlund who had sent his regards and said he would be writing to him. He wasn't surprised at Backlund's opting out of foetal work but couldn't really understand such a position. He was rather upset about the London neurologists reacting negatively to the news of his first operation which they had intended for themselves.

Now came the timing. It was no longer if, it was when. It would take a month, he said to wean me off all my drugs, which he said, should happen slowly. That would take us into July, so that I would be able to attend my son's graduation from college in June.

We left the hospital more uncertain than when we arrived. Hitchcock had not suggested I speak with any of the patients who had received the graft, and I had not found the temerity to ask. And our stated agreement to wait three months to see their results was not mentioned again. If I allowed myself to forget the excitement generated by the daily reference in the national and international press clippings, I was left with doubts and more doubts. Lili was left wondering whether she would again be dragged in as the accomplice, to give her seal of approval to something, the outcome of which she felt would be negative.

The climate for the operation was ripening. Frequently when I switched on the TV or the radio, there was some news from Birmingham with the modest, soothing voice of the professor explaining his work and how it had accidentally come to public notice. If by chance I missed it, excited friends, colleagues and tradesmen drew my attention to it, including the idea, held by the builder supervising the structural works to our house at this time, that I, like Betty Knight, might become a TV star. A very serious consideration, on the other hand, was the real fear that I might miss the opportunity if I didn't grasp at it now.

Next day, I took myself off my two drugs, Pergolide and Deprenyl, without saying anything about it. Perhaps it was my way of propelling a decision which I might have found too difficult to make. The sudden withdrawal of two of my three drugs had instant effect as the receptors went into reverse gear. I had to confess to what I could no longer conceal.

That evening, we discussed dates seriously, and I ended up attaching my decision to the holiday break from my psychotherapist. I thought it would be preferable to go up to Birmingham and have the operation while the therapist was still in London, instead of waiting for the August holidays.

The withdrawal of the drugs left me weaker and more immobile by the day. I spent more and more time in bed, reinforcing the need for the operation which, in a bold if not magical sweep, seemed a chance to correct this deficiency and release me for good from the withdrawal of drugs which I would no longer be needing.

Lili, shuddering at the memory of the other trials, summed it up by saying that I would be a guinea pig for a twenty-first century operation done on the basis of some hyped-up headlines and some results yet to be published. She also felt that, by now, I was hardly in a position to be objective about it. In truth, I was already emotionally committed to the operation.

We made an appointment to see our excellent and caring GP, Andrew Elder, who had undertaken, when we signed on with him, to curb my excesses and take some responsibility from my wife in making a decision. He, too, hadn't the heart to say no in the face of my Houdini-like determination to attempt to escape from my Parkinsonian strait-jacket.

I talked also to Drs Stern and Parkes. David Parkes was totally against it, and Gerald Stern was non-committal. He was constrained by medical ethics not to interfere and possibly a shade interested in what the outcome might be.

Uppermost in our minds was, why was I chosen among eight hundred applicants, and why could I choose my time? Was it because I was a medical colleague? Or would it be useful if it succeeded and it was reported in the press? When it was over, one newspaper later reported that the fourth patient was a doctor. So much for my ambition for stardom.

Discussion with our sons proved futile; both were preoccupied with their studies and their futures. My oldest son, Gideon, was having a hard time at art college after obtaining his degree at Cambridge. My second son, after graduating had planned a summer job in Hong Kong. Both were put out by the turmoil and uprooting from our home, while under siege from the builders.

And so the decision was taken without them and the date set for 12 June.

The day before going to Birmingham was spent in the truly magnificent surroundings of the Manoir aux Quat' Saisons, near Oxford, at the birthday celebration of a great friend of ours and my tennis partner. The minimalist portions, so tasty and artistically presented, together with the unique warmth of our Greek hosts, was a good antidote to the hospital fare ahead. The pink Cru Bourgeois Champagne and the Pouilly Fumé Les Berthiers, however, induced an excruciating migrainous headache. Back home I curled up into a deep sleep and the throbbing finally subsided.

In all the rush of next morning, I had to go to my therapist. I hadn't packed till about 11.15 a.m. A good friend insisted on driving us to Birmingham even though he had a crucial board meeting in London at 2 p.m.

We arrived at noon, this time at the proper carriage entrance to the Midlands Neurosurgery and Neurology Hospital, the new wing facing allotments and stretching into an orchard of mature, fruit-laden trees. The frequent ambulances drawing up at the entrance indicated that the centre was an acute and accident hospital, where relatives waited in the corridors for miracles which rarely happened. The grass under the plum trees remained untrodden.

The sliding doors, touched off by remote control beam, opened to an anonymous welcome. The lady behind the glass partition in the brick-faced entrance lobby sent us on our way down a series of highly polished corridors through the single-storey building to our destination in room seven. It was a private room with Venetian shutters and had a bathroom en suite. It was attached to ward ten, an acute neurological ward, and clearly the professor's own domain. We were both reminded of Pamplona, an English version of it, with TV but without religious censor.

We were hungry, and Lili went to the staff canteen, a haven which for the next three long weeks was to become a place of social encounters, information, warm support and gossip.

I was taken over by a plump, dark-eyed student nurse who was keen to take my blood pressure, temperature and pulse. She was very motherly and chatted about her visit to the dentist that morning while showing me around the facilities of the ward. She was followed by the staff nurse who spoke with a pronounced Birmingham intonation. She too spoke with warmth and openness. Then came Dr Buxton who curtly introduced himself and said he'd been 'entertaining the examiners' in Edinburgh. He examined me while looking straight ahead into the distance. On completing his examination, he outlined the treatment plan. First they would try to stabilize me on as little, or no drug at all, in order to gauge the benefit of the operation. The neurosurgeons felt that their availability three times a day to adjust dosages enabled them to obtain better observation and stability than a neurologist who only sees his patient once a week.

When all else failed to improve those conditions, then, and then only, would surgery be considered. I could see how this applied in cases of badly diagnosed and poorly assessed patients. But it didn't apply to me, with my accurate and consistent charts of the daily Ons and Offs and Inbetweens with which I arrived, as I did for all my trials.

And so, like a guinea pig in a pen, with all my medication restricted, and with all my autonomy gone, I settled back to be cared for in the hospital. My go-between was my wife who was there to protect me. I felt as if a new era was dawning, or at least, that such a possibility existed. At the same time, there were cautionary feelings that we had been there before and had been bitterly disappointed.

Prof. Hitchcock came in the late afternoon – friendly, cordial and charming. He said that the depletion of L-dopa could possibly stimulate the receptors to accept the foetal cells and that was why he intended to cut the L-dopa to zero or close to zero.

This aroused terror in my wife, from previous experience of withdrawal effects. She told the professor forcefully about the experience of removal of all drugs, and that willing subject though I was, I was not prepared to accept such a regime. He modified his prescription to as little dopamine as I could tolerate and put me on hourly doses of my own brand, dispersible Madopar, which was unavailable in the hospital pharmacy. Fortunately, I had brought a small supply and this I took until more could be obtained. He ordered a CAT scan to be done and a Nuclear Magnetic Resonance test, on an expensive and sophisticated piece of equipment owned by and operated in three centres in England, of which Coventry was the nearest. Access to the PET scan in London's Hammersmith Hospital was jealously controlled by the neurological establishment in

London and the professor was denied use of it for his graft patients at that time. The scans would reveal before and after views of the area operated on; in the case of the CAT scan, a shadow in the area would reveal the transplant.

He had heard on the grapevine that the two cases done in the joint Anglo-Swedish venture had not registered any change. He described the great simplicity of the operation and deplored the running sore of insufficient funds hampering the research. Finally, he ordered videos of me to be taken by his instrument-maker, Bill, who also dabbles in electronics. These would document motor behaviour before and after the transplantation.

The next morning sure enough, on the stage of the lecture theatre in the new wing, surrounded by a permanent display of pickled human brains with various manifestations of disease, I performed for Bill's camera. A green mop cap concealed every last strand of hair, and I walked, I stood and sat, first in an Off state, then later in an On state. A button of the gown I was wearing was left open in each series, as a clue to which state was being portrayed.

Of the many investigations to be done, there remained the lumbar puncture. For this, Mr Buxton made me curl up in a foetal position before palpating for the correct level at which to anaesthetize locally and finally, to enter the space and tap off spinal fluid. The thought that this was to be the first of a number of such probes frightened me. Having done many of these myself, I anticipated each move with apprehension, most particularly, the final thrust into the inter-vertebral space. I was relieved when a small phial of translucent liquid was produced and I despatched the nurse with it to show my wife, who had been sent outside and was anxiously waiting in the corridor, with a remark about the finely distilled gin for the evening cocktail.

I settled down to the prescribed six hours flat on my back

to avoid headache. I was free from major discomfort and passed the second night in hospital without incident.

Because of the distance to the nearest rooming house in suburban Birmingham, and the need to keep an eye on the builders, Lili decided to commute on alternate nights. For the rest, a folding camp bed was found for her by the nurses, with permission to use the floor space in my room.

Fraught with the logistics of protecting our belongings from the builders who were not only dismantling our house but discontinuing all services in the process; martialling the children and keeping an eye on what was going on with me, Lili returned next afternoon. Together we went on a tour of the surroundings, a veritable small corner of Pakistan and much the livelier for it. Lili was excited by the display of fabrics and the ladies in bright trouser suits and shawls, imaginatively assembled, sitting chatting at the counters with the store keepers of the open-fronted stores. After the post-lumbar puncture confinement, it was a relief to get out of the hospital. Lili reminded me that most people go to hospital to get better. Me, I went to hospital to get ill.

My next interview was with Dr Hughes, the consultant neurologist in the project. His sober and realistic approach to my undergoing the operation reawakened some doubts about it, especially when he pointed to the limited improvement which might be expected. We discussed another drug being experimentally used at the Middlesex Hospital for the past two years. It is called Apomorphine, an agonist like the Pergolide I was using for treating the oscillations. Because it was being injected subcutaneously, and with the spectre of Pamplona in mind, I had mixed feelings about it and never made a formal request to be on the trial. After talking to Dr Hughes, about the operation it seemed a reasonable alternative, especially when viewed from a position of being Off, when often everything seems hopeless.

The artificial excitement generated in the beginning was

now over and the quiet reality and decision-making remained. Lili spent the night on the camp bed in my room, but neither of us got much sleep. I had great difficulty in turning over in the hospital bed; there was a wide swathe of light above the ward door, and the nurses chattered loudly all night at their station, relying on heavily sedated patients to be beyond disturbance. The stories they related and the giggling went on until dawn and I thought longingly of my electric bed at home.

We had a Sunday morning visit from Prof. Hitchcock, who drove up from his Worcestershire home in the country to visit. He came in, his arms crossed on his slender chest, and he listened attentively to my account of the interview with Dr Hughes.

We had a leisurely talk during which he expressed his disappointment in the medical establishment. He acknowledged the inevitability of professional competition, 'but a little nod of acknowledgement from my colleagues would be in order, don't you think?' He was referring to the fact that all British neurologists had studiously avoided any recognition or reference to his pioneering operation in this country. As to the time of my operation, the decision was with the neurologist, who, in his capacity as assessor, was to decide when I was ready. 'I am just as keen as you are for an early resolution to your PD', he said, 'but we must be patient'.

He explained the presence of a neurologist on his transplant programme in order to establish a base line assessment. He summarily dismissed the Apomorphine. How could one go around continuously injecting one's own system! On the other hand, he had no answer to the question of *why* his surgical patients had shown a slight initial improvement. Embryonic cells are mysterious, he said.

He mentioned that the Parkinson's Disease Society had been approached by the BBC to make an in-depth film about the operation, to which he had no objection. Lili, hoping to avoid my having to undergo more lumbar punctures and knowing of the available alternative at the Hammersmith Hospital, had rung a neurologist there whom I knew. He was one of the team with access to the PET scan and could inquire whether Prof. Hitchcock's patients, and specifically I, could use it. The answer had been a categorical *no*. When she reported this to the professor, he was shocked and shook his head in dismay and puzzlement.

He said that the BMA wanted a government-appointed medical team to issue guidelines for the foetal graft; the Polkinghorne Committee finally made its recommendations exactly a year later. His personal guideline was, that if medication is inadequate to control the condition, surgery is indicated.

This conversation showed how preoccupying were the ethical and political considerations belabouring the whole process since the story broke wide open with Hitchcock's first operation in April. Hates and jealousies sometimes abounded, I felt, ignoring the crying need of Parkinson's patients. On the other hand, this *was* a relatively untried procedure and could be premature, at the very least, and disappointing.

Over lunch in the canteen where Lili chatted with staff, the buzz was all about the operation on Betty, which had propelled the active, but unknown 'Neuro', as the hospital was referred to by bus drivers and shopkeepers in the Birmingham area, into the nation's headlines and fame. The electrician bore witness to the great improvement: 'You should have seen her walk down the corridor!' he said, referring to the outpatients' department where previously she had been wheeled in. A Korean neurosurgeon, also at lunch, had come to observe the professor's technique, and was hoping that I would be ready for such an observation before he had to return home.

To pass the inert time that hangs heavily on hospitals on Sundays, we set out to go into Birmingham to visit the art gallery. The day was bright and sunny and the clouds were racing across the blue sky over the allotments below. We waited in vain for a bus that never came, then walked down to Smethwick. Skirting the road were more prosperous semi-detached houses with neatly tended sloping front gardens. All roads were winding and seemed endlessly long. At the bottom of the hill, where the bearded elders of the community were holding their counsel, leaning turbaned heads on sticks and nodding, I said goodbye to my wife, because time had run out for her to return to New Street station and London.

The next day, while Lili was home rescuing plants in my consulting room from the heavy plaster work, the professor came into my room and hinted obliquely that the surgical solution to my Parkinson's disease was now in order. I could not quite understand and never discovered what had so moved him into a positive view. Had the neurologist completed his observations for the base line to satisfy the Ethical Committee of the hospital, or was he merely following a form of protocol to satisfy all? I did know, however, that my doubts had dispersed, and I had a vision of a grafted cell, multiplying constantly to complement my own inadequate system, secreting a steady level of dopamine, and that I would feel restored.

Now that I had made up my mind, I was impatient, and, with the minimal dosage of Madopar I was allowed, very parkinsonian and uncomfortable. I was Off most of the day, becoming akinetic, as the paltry store of dopamine diminished. It was the equivalent of a drug holiday. I tried to escape the extreme heat of my room and went to sit under a lovely copper Prunus tree in the orchard, which reminded me of the one in our front garden at home. But it didn't help. Even when Lili came back from London with lots of cheery cards and my favourite pastries from the Swiss shop in St John's Wood, my mood did not improve.

CHAPTER 15

The Operation

I had had to vacate my room for a private patient of the professor, 'she's paying', he'd apologetically said, referring to the chronic and inhibiting lack of funds dogging his transplant research, with all fees from private patients going into the kitty.

The new room had a door leading into the main ward, with a concave, two-way functioning mirror in the corner at ceiling level, monitoring me and enabling me to watch the action in the ward. It had no bathroom and the floor space for the camp bed was restricted.

When the professor came to see me that day, he said the

only thing holding up the operation now was the go-ahead from Dr Hughes. He told me that he would be looking for a suitable embryo tomorrow, because if the graft could not be done in the next two days there would be a longish delay as he was not available for stereotactic surgery.

I had found out how it would happen. A phone call from a nursing home twenty minutes away from the hospital would alert the professor and his team that a termination of pregnancy was about to happen. He then delegates his duties, where possible, and rushes over to personally perform the delicate task of dissecting the striatal embryonic cells. He places these in a culture and brings it back in a portable refrigerator, in readiness for transplantation.

Meantime, I would be prepared for the operating theatre. I slept fitfully. We were both woken up again by the echoing laughter of a cluster of nurses. Near the nurses' station and under their scrutiny, a man lay dying. His distraught wife was walking around the bed in shocked disbelief, full of tears and clutching the cup of tea the nurses had kindly thrust into her rigid hand.

Her husband, I learnt later, a man in his fifties, had been painting his house that sunny afternoon and fallen off the ladder. Despite the skill of the surgeons, he had fought and lost his battle. How devastating for the family to lose their father so pointlessly. I tried to comfort Lili who had no experience of hospital wards with their sudden deaths, and fell into a fitful sleep.

I woke up that morning with a great deal of anticipation hoping that today might be the day. The morning was a dull and misty Midlands morning with little visibility across the hospital boundary. I washed and dressed and tidied up. I was beginning to find it hard to live a life and leave space for the nurses' tasks. I tried my best to keep my small amenity room in order - my books, tapes, medication, greetings cards and journals were disposed of in the coded plastic sacks which linked their colour to the hierarchy of disposal.

I knew the patient had died when the nurses came to close the door opening onto the corridor. It was followed by the soft thuds which closed all the other ward doors. The passage of death is private to other candidates, and the shrouded bed passed quickly through the line of curtained screens that were aligned in its passage. It was a ritual which, as young hospital doctors, we left to the nurses and one I became familiar with in this hospital in the days to come.

The ward round that morning was led by Mr Kenny, the professor's senior registrar on the team. Trailing along were four wooden-looking personnel who displayed little interest or enthusiasm. The visit was a formality, the charts scrutinized briefly, and the planned visit to Coventry for the NMR scan spoken about. There was no reflection in the group of the excitement I was experiencing, or the feeling that, as a candidate for a pioneering surgical experiment, I was human under the skin. Mr Kenny did say that no cells were anticipated that day and we should go as arranged to Coventry.

We were taken by ambulance to the Walsgrave Hospital, near Coventry, but the prized machinery wasn't quite functioning and we sat in the entrance of the department for three hours waiting for it to be repaired. Outside on the grass verge, the two jolly ambulance men were luckier; they were accumulating overtime with a snooze in the sunshine. While waiting, we called ward ten to find out from sister whether on the off chance, the material had arrived. She told us it hadn't, and I had to reconcile myself to a further week's wait, with a weekend in between.

The repair of the Nuclear Magnetic Scan machine was completed. I was stretched on a mobile unit and my head passed into a tunnel. Grinding, rumbling sounds enveloped my head. I came home with plates of many coloured images that looked like a skyline at night. I had no idea how to read them and merely delivered them to Sister. A scorching headache developed on the way back in the ambulance. These had a regularity about them but on the positive side, there is nothing quite like the post-headache relief that follows it.

The remaining days of the week, without hope of action, passed with tedium and anxiety. I had another video taken in the Off phase, performing, once again, in my surgical disguise. Lili stayed with me but learnt on the telephone that the disruption at home was worse than ever and that once again our seventeen-year-old daughter had to be billeted out.

There was another terminal case of an Asian girl dying on the other side of my wall. Day and night for three nights the entire family had stayed holding vigil, the beards growing denser, the sari suits limper. But they remained until the life-support machine was switched off.

My great solace was the stodgy steam puddings drowned in custard served with comforting regularity.

On Thursday morning Prof. Hitchcock on his rounds agreed to my going home for the weekend. 'No use in institutionalizing him', he said to Lili. We leapt out, carrying the dirty laundry.

Domestic torment awaited us at home. The temporary kitchen we had been using was now dismantled; there was little space, in a small dusty area of the house, for us to use. Friends came to call. I was feeling a bit of a fraud, as two weeks had passed and I had little to show for the time spent away. I felt purposeless and became more withdrawn and distant. This only exacerbated the tense atmosphere in the house, compounded by the omnipresent workmen and the indiscriminate plaster dust everywhere.

We celebrated my son's birthday with a cake no one wanted to eat. Lili had begun to have severe worries about the whole enterprise and tried to alert me to its inconsistencies which she had observed during her stay at the neurological hospital. She was particularly fearful that I was again being used as a guinea pig; that we had seen no one who had had the operation before me, despite the fact that after being discharged, they all came back for check-ups in the outpatients' department, and brief meetings with them would have been the simplest of enterprises.

Also, she noted they seemed to have so little knowledge of the On-Off situation and what affects it, and the gross effect of drug withdrawal which constitutes a near drug holiday which all Parkinson's sufferers know to treat with utmost caution; and that the nurses without exception were untrained in and unfamiliar with basic PD assessment. They seemed to lack the experience of the wide range of mood swings and motor differences in response to the drug. They expected predictable results from L-dopa tablets as from all other medication they dispensed, unaware that the time of day, the connection between doses, the contents of the stomach and other factors influence this response. The record sheets they were required to fill in had little scope for these subtleties.

Most of all, we both wondered whether the improvement claimed in the early cases was due to a mis-diagnosis rather than successful treatment, or even the resumption of medication or stimulating briefly the cells deprived of their medication. But I had already committed two weeks to the experiment, and silenced any doubts about the competence of the people into whose hands I had delivered myself.

I left the house with a feeling of catastrophe about it, my family without a base of togetherness, and returned to the hospital early on Monday morning. Lili followed at midday, bringing her bicycle for use around the neighbourhood.

On Tuesday morning when I washed myself, I felt I was preparing for some important, if unknown, event. Confirmation of my intuition came with sister telling me I was not to have any breakfast. This surprised me, as I knew the operation was to be done under local anaesthetic. But I assumed that even done in this way, accidents requiring general anaesthetics are best avoided.

Then a young blonde secretary came with a consent form for me to sign. The professor had warned me that if I were to read it, I would probably be frightened off, and that to satisfy legal requirements it was 'ridiculous'. I didn't read it, Lili signed it screwing up her face.

News came through that the professor had the material from the histologist, but that the mother had not yet signed the consent. Anyway, the hospital scan was broken and would probably not be ready for use. The operation today would be unlikely. 'No use going into it half cocked' Hitchcock said, popping his head round the door. 'I'll say', I remember thinking wryly. He sat down in his chummy manner, crossing his arms, and, addressing me in the urbane, collegiate manner of a fellow physician, he raised the matter of where to place the foetal cells when he got them. All three previous grafts had been placed in the caudate nucleus. A new site, the putamen, which had never before been used for a graft on apes or man, carried a greater risk because of deeper penetration, but recent research had shown that the putamen was the site most affected by the disease. In response to Lili's question 'how deep?', he responded by describing a distance of about two inches between his forefinger and his thumb. In his reckoning, the risk factor increased from 0.5 per cent to two per cent, of haemorrhage, or stroke or both. On the other hand, it might have a better chance of success. In any case he was keen to try if I were game enough.

It was thrown out as a challenge, and with the confidence backed by his supreme and internationally acknowledged skill as a stereotactic surgeon. He breezed out not awaiting my reply saying he'd come back later to hear my decision.

Sitting on a chair across the room, Lili was appalled. She expressed her revulsion against such an untried and almost cavalier approach to what might have long-lasting and irreversible effects. I was tempted to go all the way. We argued a long time. I never said yea or nay.

It was at lunchtime when we were chatting with a fellow PD sufferer from Birmingham University, that the door flung open and Mr Kenny rushed in, brushing everyone aside and said 'Right, you're on!' I felt the colour drain from my face. I had waited for this moment for so long, but wasn't really prepared for it at this time. Kenny told Lili to take a long walk and went to work on me.

He put me into a barber's chair, tied a huge sheet around me and with this improvisation and an unsophisticated electric razor that alternately cut and pulled, shaved off all my hair. When, accompanied by many tired wisecracks, my head was shaven clean, he injected local anaesthetic and drilled four holes into my skull in order to attach to it the foot-square stainless steel frame designed by Bill, the technical expert. The great moment had arrived and whereas before it was all conjecture and theory, we were now into brain surgery, whatever name it went by.

It felt very 'space age'. He draped a green surgical cloth around the whole. There was a long and uncomfortable wait. With the structure on my head I couldn't relax or recline and just sat stiff and upright marking the hours. At last, at 3.45 p.m., I was wheeled into the X-ray department for a CAT scan which had been repaired just in time to assist with targeting the chosen area.

I was still pondering fifty-fifty about where I wanted the graft to be placed, with a strong bias towards the putamen, the riskier but more hopeful site. Another hour passed and Hitchcock and Kenny came in. All is ready, said the

Professor, except the HIV test 'unless you wouldn't mind a small dose of AIDS'. I didn't fall about laughing, instead, I took some medication which the nurses had forgotten to give me. The professor said about one and a half hours to go. I was put into a white gown, and then the yellow sports shirt I was wearing wouldn't pass over my head gear, so some scissors had to be found to slit it open and remove it.

Time passed me. Images of McEnroe playing for his seeding position floated in and out of my vision. Lili tried to continue interesting me in the Mahler biography, from which I had earlier read her a description of his passionate conducting.

The professor asked me whether I had made my decision. To Lili's horror I replied, 'you decide, just don't tell me about it'. 'Caudate nucleus as before it is,' he said, tripping out swiftly in his medical school tie and blazer, Kenny respectfully hovering by his side.

At 6.20 p.m. a green-coated theatre nurse and a porter came and wheeled me down the corridors to the theatre where the surgeon and the team were waiting. I was transferred to a very narrow operating table, my head frame was attached to the apparatus that secured the stereo. Behind me, on both sides were lit-up screens against which the X-rays were displayed. Everything happened very quickly or so, after all the waiting, it seemed. A saline drip was introduced into my right arm in case of emergencies. In the event, it was used only for a prophylactic antibiotic.

I saw the professor going over to a trolley on which stood the jar containing the material and drew some of it up into a syringe. They drilled a hole through my front skull and it reminded me of having an upper molar drilled at the dentist, only this time no one suggested that I open wide. Not much was said, only Hitchcock and Kenny suggesting the right angles for the injection carrying the foetal cells to the intended place. Nor was I aware of the actual placement of the foetal cells. I had a great sense of unreality and had to actually remind myself this was happening to me.

It was nearly over and the skin over the hole, the size of a five pence piece, was sutured and dressed. The frame was removed and the wounds from the attachment to the frame were treated. I was directing my attention to the noises emanating from my head, wondering what differences might be taking place. The conjectured dreams of nearly a decade had been realized and I wondered whether, and when, there would be some benefits.

In the most poignant moment of the procedure, the professor thanked me for trusting him. For the rest, it was back on the rolling bed in which I was whisked back to my room. I do not know how long I was gone. Still anaesthetized, I did not feel the pain that my ashen-faced wife perceived when I was delivered back. She thought that my head looked like a football that had been kicked around. The professor, re-dressed in civilian clothes came by and remarked 'at least we haven't made him worse', no doubt referring to the hazards he had outlined.

From then on I felt that my condition justified my being in intensive care. The nurses went into their familiar post-operative routine with efficiency. In addition to recording my pulse and blood pressure, they checked my reflexes, my accommodation to light and overall alertness. The professor came back at ten o'clock in the evening. Dr Clough came later, and so did Mr Kenny. All inspected the goods with satisfaction.

For me the drilling had been the worst part, and now my head was beginning to throb with pain under the tight bandage.

Lili filled a catheter bag from the nurses' trolley with ice and put it over my head, but despite this I had a bad night and a full-blown migraine in the morning. It came with a heavy feeling and pain in my abdomen and I wondered whether I had developed some allergy to the coloured dye injected into my veins for the scan. Lili was worried because I must have given the impression of some urgency. She fetched the duty doctor who, after examining me, reassured me it was not the spleen, or the liver, but old-fashioned constipation. A suppository was prescribed and took effect the next day, and I felt some relief.

On the second day, the professor came in the morning and ripped off the bandage which gave me further relief. For the first time we saw the holes in the skull, drilled to hold the cage, and the wound with its stitches. The CAT scan post-operatively showed nothing untoward, Mr Kenny reported, just a little swelling from the graft. Just a shadow over my brain. The professor said it is nothing at all, just to see the graft is there. They were both pleased with a job well done.

I now joined the ranks of the convalescents, the men and women in dressing gowns and green caps. The summer weather was beguiling. We sat on the lawns onto which the wards opened up and spilt out their mobile patients. The professor called it a holiday camp, as he sped by and quipped 'some people are lucky!' But the light was too strong and I preferred the enclosure and darkness of my room.

Taking her cue from my stomach upset, Lili went off on her bicycle in search of fresh vegetables and roughage which were hard to find in the nearby corner sweet shops. She returned with a red cabbage, carrots and cauliflower, which she chopped up with the butter knife and gave me to eat out of a plastic pill dish.

I still felt unwell and depressed. The following day was Rafael's graduation day at Cambridge, and although I knew missing it had been a calculated risk, when the day came, I felt very disappointed. In London, the builders awaited settlement of their due amount and Lili had to arrange the banking and meeting on site before going to Cambridge to attend graduation. She caught an evening train. I felt nauseous and vomited several times. When I felt better, I walked around the hospital and took stock.

When Lili came back, after meandering around East Anglia on an impossible train connection from Cambridge to Birmingham, with an account of the age-old ceremony which I had already experienced with our eldest son, I had turned the corner to recovery. Although I still tired easily, we went on outings between ward rounds and tried to imagine what the future might hold with the benefits of the foetal cells providing drive and motivation. I began to distance myself from involvement with the ward inhabitants and the nurses with their problems, and to conserve emotional energy for the return to my family and my patients.

This was not easy, as our home was still a building site with no access to the bedroom and no kitchen facilities. Repairs to the flank wall involved half the house vertically and there was little space in which to exist. Lili went to see off our son to Hong Kong and ascertained that for a while at least we couldn't go home.

I had planned a meeting of a small group of fellow Parkinson's sufferers who meet regularly in our home during the year. They are contemporary in age and profession and all interested in transplant as a treatment of the future. A special impetus was the visit to England of Sidney Dorros, a Parkinsonian who has been active in organizing self-help groups all over the United States. I hoped to help raise funds required by the professor to continue his project in the future.

The meeting convened in the lecture theatre on 29 June at noon. At nine o'clock that morning, the professor came in, looked at me and said 'You can go home'. I felt a tremendous relief, compounded with concern about where we were going to be living, and excitement at the prospect of the reunion with my friends who were arriving from Bristol, Manchester, Cambridge and Birmingham. They had all arrived and were waiting in the conference room where the kitchen staff had laid out a spread of tasty sandwiches and pots of coffee next to the cakes Lili had brought from London.

Seated around the large conference table the professor, in his white coat, outlined, with great clarity, the history of his transplant programme. He would have preferred, he said, to get on with it without media attention. I had intended to relate my experience of the operation, but when the time came I was Off and exhausted. This was a real disappointment and I had to go and lie down in my room instead. At 5.15 p.m. my drugs arrived from the pharmacy, we said our good-byes to the nursing staff, and we were ready to go, still not having made any arrangements where to go. The professor repeated his thanks to me for trusting him to do the operation. Then, for the last time, he went through his teaching routine of leaning his head sideways with arms akimbo, looking at me, his patient, turning to the assembled ward round of senior registrar, houseman, sister, nurse and, in this case, his secretary: 'I don't want to say it, but what do you think?' A chorus of approval came back with: 'Much more expression, better smile', everyone noticed an improvement.

I had a big stake in their obedient optimism. For months I, my family and friends scrutinized my features, and, as time passed, knew the futility of hope for which there was no basis in reality.

With pills in my pocket and a sailor's cap on my head we and the bicycle left the hospital in a taxi headed for the nearest Holiday Inn.

CHAPTER 16

For Better or Worse

By electing to undergo the operation in Birmingham, I had effectively broken the established links with my neurological carers in London.

It was their repeated delays and the over-cautiousness about the ethical considerations in their approach to trying out transplant research that had frustrated me and in the end led me to approach Prof. Hitchcock in Birmingham.

When the London neurologists did move in a joint effort with the Swedish group from Lund, they delayed announcing the results of their joint venture till a year had passed. To me that had seemed too long. Although the brave attempt of pioneers throughout American centres and Birmingham would seem to have been premature, some unknown frontier had been crossed for the future, and all people plagued with Parkinson's disease were roused from hopeless inertia to a sense of expectation.

The coincidence of the rebuilding of our house and the Birmingham operation left us stranded for one week without a home base. We made out way down to London in slow stages, passing through Stratford where we saw a Restoration play. In the first row of the Swan Theatre my tremor was so gross that for the first time, for fear of impeding the concentration of people sitting behind me, I removed myself to the back row of the theatre. We had a picnic of the best of Marks & Spencer supplies on the banks of the Avon and threw the leftovers to the ducks. The week ended with a stay in Aldeburgh, where we settled down to the idyllic sound of the breakers on the pebble shore below our window. It didn't last. The sound of hammering and sawing soon intruded into the peace. The builders were there, too. The hotel was taking the end-of-season opportunity to build new bathrooms on the floor above. So we hastened home, where I hired a consulting room nearby while our house was being completed, and shuttled to the top floor to see my patients.

I wandered through the recovery period wearing a Basque beret to crown my surgical baldness. The hole in the head healed rapidly and without complication. I was sensitive to any changes in behaviour or emanations from my head, looking for signs to be interpreted as indications of growth of foetal cells. The most hopeful sign, in the first three months, was an awareness of a throbbing at the back of my head, usually around midnight before going to sleep.

Whatever sounds or pulsations there were, there was no shift in behaviour or ease of movement. When On, I felt less encumbered than before the operation; when Off, I dipped lower and had less resource to sustain myself than before. I had too little time On and felt too sluggish to work more than a few hours in the morning and one in the evening, with no option but to rest helplessly all afternoon. A short walk round the block was my sole exercise. Social life was very restricted and theatre and concert life a rarity. I was simply too tired at night and much of the day. I had not really taken into account the fact that I had undergone brain surgery, as well as being without two component parts of my medication and still experiencing withdrawal symptoms from one of them, the Pergolide.

There was a growing sense of disappointment as the months ticked by. Hopes had been high that the operation would be successful. I had reckoned for myself that if one was seeking a cure, uncomplicated by side effects, it would have to come by operation rather than by replacement chemistry. Transplanted material was more likely to secrete the whole spectrum of chemical elements that would make up deficits, including those that still await discovery.

I returned to the hospital at three-month and six-month intervals. Despite the professor's encouragement and his exhortation not to 'let him down', my hopes were beginning to dwindle by this time. He insisted that the others in the series were doing 'so well'. Since there was such a drop in my own performance from before the operation, when I was taking the Pergolide, I made a special journey to see if I could start up the Pergolide again. Hitchcock agreed to adding only the Deprenyl but felt anything more would invalidate the experiment.

When I could no longer tolerate the brevity of span of active life which the On provided, I once again took the train to Birmingham with Lili. It was a gloomy damp December day. We had a long depressing wait in the familiar corridors of the hospital. It was my last visit, and my last meeting with the professor, because when we persuaded the neurologist and the professor that I needed some chemical help to make life tolerable, he reluctantly agreed to my resuming the support agonist and sadly dismissed me from the research programme. I had ceased to be number four.

I had braced myself against feelings that the operation might fail or, even worse, that I might lose some of my own irreplaceable brain cells. The first line of defence was penetrated initially by the check-up after three months, when there was no benefit to be recognized. There was a discrepancy between the professor's optimism and my experience. I argued against my negativism by saying I was always trying to be ahead of myself and the happening, but in my observations of my body functions nothing contradicted my feeling that the graft was not secreting dopamine.

My thought processes had slowed down even when the Madopar was being effective. My family noticed that I paused over my answers, my conversation lacked spontaneity, and I found myself posturing to overcome the fumbling for speedier reply and a better flow of conversation. In part the bradyphrenia, the slow thinking, was a result of Parkinson's disease, but whereas that used to respond to medication early in the day, it was no longer the case. My feelings seemed to be all frozen over. I was depressed and disappointed.

I felt that having the operation when I did was premature and an ill-considered risk. I had been so excited to be selected from such a large pool of candidates that I had put aside my cautious judgment, failing to elicit answers to the obvious questions concerning animal studies replicating the operation and to request a detailed study of just how the three earlier candidates had been assessed before and after. I had doubts about their assessment of me. Just what was being sought beyond an undefined sense of improvement, not clearly a consequence of the graft? To be directly related to the graft, the improvement would have to be greater on the side opposite the graft, following the neurological pathways. This had not happened in my case.

Holding on to the inflated hope that maintained an image of perfection in action was only to be obtained from a graft operation, I had obscured what was actually happening with the graft, and just how minimal the benefits were for the person seen on TV, as opposed to the written words and big headlines in the press. This position of mine involved self-delusion in which I was both the successful surgeon and the patient as the triumphant collaborator. It was as if it were all a sequence on film rather than a real happening.

One evening in winter I bumped into Gerald Stern before a performance of *The Tempest* at the Old Vic. 'It didn't work, did it?' he said, taking one look at my pale haggard face. I was forced to agree. When he added, 'come and have a chat', I felt free to join, once more, the Thursday morning coffee breaks attended by his students and registrars.

I started taking Pergolide in February. The effect was instant and expectable. I had long Ons and was looking forward to a better quality of life again, when about four weeks later, I had a heart attack followed by a near fatal cardiac arrest.

CHAPTER 17

Cardiac Arrest

An unexpected event prodded my memory of this near-death experience, which made all others seem insignificant. Our house guest from America, the same friend who had come to my family's rescue when I was hospitalized at the Royal Free Hospital fifteen years ago, had been successfully treated for lung cancer and had enjoyed her two-week visit with us to celebrate her recovery. The day before leaving, she coughed up three thimblesful of bright red blood. I quickly arranged for her to be seen at St Mary's Hospital. We drove her there and our route was a familiar one; I found myself in the same cubicle that I had occupied when, on a gusty Saturday evening in March, I was delivered there, and collapsed unconscious on the same bed. I had no recall of the event. But I remembered that I had experienced a tightness under the breastbone from early in the morning. I had been having mild indigestion for some days, dousing myself with antacid tablets.

My daughter was performing a solo violin in a recital at the Guildhall School of Music, a sort of run-through for her final term performance with the orchestra at St Paul's School. I was very keen to hear this and put the pain out of my mind, thinking that I'd get round to the casualty department for an electrocardiogram sometime that day. I ask myself now why I was so indifferent about it. The closest I could come to an answer was that I was getting increasingly depressed with the emerging awareness of the failure of the operation.

When deeply depressed, I felt isolated and found it difficult to talk, which in turn added to the isolation. Delaying seeking help may then have been an expression of a wish to be rid of it all – many years of illness and battling had left me depleted and empty.

I have since been told by cardiologists that doctors usually procrastinate in the face of chest pains, assuming that it is indigestion.

I came home from the concert and sat quietly sipping water. A colleague and friend, whom my wife had contacted while waiting for our GP to come, kept me company. Hours passed while we sat. After three hours the answering service finally made a connection and a young woman duty doctor arrived, embarrassed by the inefficiency of the service. The combination of a slow pulse and the tight pain in the chest, left her in no doubt that I should have an ECG.

She offered to order an ambulance, which I declined. A taxi arrived after a further delay and dropped us about fifty yards from the entrance of the new wing at St Mary's Hospital. We walked the remainder of the way.

I was seen immediately. In the cubicle, the ECG machine wasn't working. When it finally did function and a clear reading was taken, it showed that the pulse-rate was low enough for the technicians to summon the registrar.

The last thing I remember is beckoning my wife and whispering in her ear, 'It isn't indigestion'. This comment was intended to have a touch of the humour of the gallows. Then I keeled over backwards on to the bed in the cubicle. I have no recollection of the alarm ringing to summon the resuscitation team as they wheeled me into the high-tech room, equipped for such emergencies. My wife was alone and tremendously shocked, having walked into the hospital with me. They told her that my heart had stopped and I wasn't breathing and asked her to summon relatives. They offered her a cup of tea and gave her a coin for the telephone. As it was Saturday night, all the children were at parties and unreachable.

The skill of the staff and their teamwork saved me, and when they allowed Lili into the resuscitation room I just kept asking what had happened, having no recollection of events.

She was enormously relieved, but was told that the next forty-eight hours were the crucial ones. I was wheeled to the four-bed coronary care unit in the old building and looked after by a New Zealand supply nurse, who combined great nursing skill with emotional support. Prof. Sheridan, most courteously, broke his Sunday rest and came to supervise my diagnosis and treatment.

When I got better, I was told that the Pergolide I had reinstated six weeks earlier might be implicated in the production of an arrhythmia; so I would have to do without the additional dopamine agonist as it was thought that

Pergolide and other dopamine agonists all potentially have that effect. But then, so does L-dopa.

My comfortable recovery was coloured by the sudden withdrawal of this drug which had so improved the quality of my daily life. The only pain I had was from my bruised ribcage, which was caused by the pressure applied on the chest to restart the heart, and from the electrodes they had used. The heart didn't falter again, and I was moved to the elegant new building which was more in line with the modern casualty department, whose alertness had saved my life. I was a genuine patient at last, with an acute problem like others around me, not someone seeking the attention, often in a very masochistic way and for the wrong reasons, as had often been the case before. Also friends could visit me near my home, unlike Pamplona, Vienna or Birmingham. People can identify with a heart attack in a way that isn't the case with Parkinson's disease. The main difference was yet to come. Having survived the heart attack I could be rehabilitated and lead an active life. PD is a chronic condition; for someone who has experienced years of treatment, an acute life-threatening illness is of a different order. A sense of release followed my recovery.

On my discharge, Prof. Sheridan suggested I participate in a rehabilitation group based in St Charles' Hospital. Since I was not allowed to work for six weeks anyway, I gave myself over to the recommended programme.

This was an open-ended group of suitable post-cardiac patients, who gathered in a Portakabin in the crowded hospital grounds for two hours three times a week, over a period of seven weeks. My exercise tolerance when tested before beginning was quite good. I had no further angina since that first Saturday. Under the discriminating and enjoyable tutorship of the senior physiotherapist, Belinda Hobbs, we limbered up, jumped on the trampoline, threw a heavy medicine ball, walked up and down steps and skipped with a rope, as well as walking on the treadmill.

Everyone learned to take their pulse before and after. Breathless, but relaxed, we all then adjourned next door to our lecture discussions on food intake, diet, recognition and avoidance of stress, fear and insecurity after a heart attack. The mixed-class group worked well. Initially, I was aware of a problem of communicating. But this didn't prevent me from working hard at the first half of the programme of exercises and breaking the defensive barrier I had set around myself. In the discussion which followed, this was reinforced. Whereas at first I thought it too big a commitment, I looked forward to each session with pleasure and was cycling the three miles in the early morning to the hospital.

It was interesting to note the growth that took place in the group. People participating quickly became familiar with the routine and assumed supportive roles to new members in the same way they had been supported when they first joined. As for me, I was pleased for the first time to be a patient rather than being a Parkinsonian and a psychotherapeutic patient.

Instead, I listened with fresh understanding to the illustrations of stress introduced and explained by the psychologist and felt better for it. I listened seriously and for the first time, to the excellent advice of the dietician, with every intention of changing my ways. Most of all, among the craftsmen, workmen and businessmen, no one singled me out as suffering from a chronic illness. They took my reticence for professional quietness, and a need in my work to listen rather than talk. Most of all, they accepted me without question as one of the group, sharing their problems and their cures.

CHAPTER 18

A Fresh Start

The cardiac arrest shocked me into a fresh awareness of the physical neglect of my body since the transplant operation, nearly a year earlier. Because of the continuous depression that had absorbed me, I had spent a large portion of my time resting and waiting in vain for some positive indication of the success of the operation. I had a schedule of exercises for Parkinson's disease patients which, because these were done alone, I carried out irregularly. I was aware of the absence of a supervisor to instil some order into the routine and some motivation for persistence.

I had stopped my personal psychotherapy in July 1988,

and felt that the termination left much to be desired. Nevertheless, I was determined to keep the agreed ending day. My disappointment in not working out something helpful in the psychotherapy of the mind-body relationship was considerable. It was at this point that I decided to approach the mind-body in the other direction, namely to explore the body as a centre of treatment.

My participation in the hospital rehabilitation pro-gramme made me really see for myself the enormous benefit of exercise under guidance. When the hospital sessions came to an end after the prescribed seven-week term, I looked around for some way of continuing supervised exercises. A very good friend invited me to try out Popmobility in her lounge which she clears out twice a week for the purpose. The supervisor, Ken Woolcott, a former athletics coach, is an inspired teacher, sensitive to the subtleties of movement and the special needs of his pupils. He pinpoints the parts of the body which are not coordinated or moving normally and introduces exercises to correct these, in the relaxed atmos-phere of slow therapeutic music. As these movements improve, a second stage of slightly faster strong-beat music is introduced to encourage response and coordination of levers. The third stage, one of infectious and bouncy music, is brought in to motivate confidence in moving about. Since beginning these exercises, I have found that I am moving muscles which would otherwise be neglected. This is particularly beneficial in the shoulder area where stiffness of the neck refers pain to the shoulder. I enjoy much greater physical fitness in general.

I felt that music therapy would help to get to the emotional core better than words alone. I began to inquire about this relatively new form of treatment. My GP suggested a music therapist working at the holistic centre at St Marylebone Church. I was introduced to Margaret Lobo, who was very enthusiastic about the holistic approach, using singing based on the diaphragm to produce support for the voice. The therapy aimed to make one more aware of that support system. She made an impact on me as a very kind and competent person and saw the lesson as a reciprocation – she would learn from my experience of Parkinson's disease over the years and, in turn, I would benefit from her vast experience as a singer and a teacher.

In addition she had a music therapist linked to her who was over from Germany for six months on a scholarship. He geared his lesson more to rhythm as expressed in the use of drums, xylophone and piano, creating a dialogue in sound. This would transcend the physical barriers set by Parkinson's disease. I found myself anticipating these weekly sessions with relish, which was partly due to my active enjoyment of working together in close companionship with another person of a different discipline. The sheer pleasure of being free to make as much noise as I wanted to, whether on drums, or better, by voice, went some considerable way to relieving depression.

This dimension for Parkinson's sufferers, removed from their own effective voice by a combination of personal and social inertia, should be readily available for them; the alternative is to languish in a state of depression, removed from their own personal sounds. When asked about Parkinsonians' relative lack of speech in social situations, I feel that this is a complicated interaction in which the Parkinsonian, not being heard, is not listened to and so he or she abandons efforts to break through this barrier. An on-going conversation presents difficulties. The sound of one's own voice as it diminishes in such situations becomes more unfamiliar and, instead of speaking up and joining in, one tends to withdraw into listening. Such isolation should not be allowed to further devastate already circumscribed lives, and making music with others under guidance is increasingly available to counteract this.

This combination of group exercise, singing, drumming and Popmobility helped to get me over the depression I had carried with me since the Birmingham operation. My increased mobility and vocal functioning have gone a long way to overcoming the core depression I discussed in another chapter and, hopefully, altering the prognosis of the illness.

CHAPTER 19

Somatopsychic

I continued to strive to make sense of my Parkinson's disease through psychosomatic theory, but had at the same time neglected the converse, somatopsychic which had equal, if not greater, relevance to my condition. The mind's reaction to the changed body and the impact on the body image is considerable and as important as the effects produced by the mind on the body.

In Parkinson's disease this altered body image is experienced through the effects of the illness on posture, gait, handwriting and, ultimately, on self-expression – all the effects of premature ageing. This has to be fought in order to preserve self-esteem and an ego in danger of being fragmented.

I watched the development of the illness from a minor disability to one which now effectively prevents me from carrying on my profession and threatens me with increased immobility. Far from being a linear progression that one might suppose from reading about the illness, it is more of an emotional rollercoaster that one learns to negotiate or rather, one takes the ride knowing there is no alternative. The variation in behaviour is more usefully compared with the development of a musical composition with its highs and lows, repetition and development of themes.

The capacity to respond positively to the medication supports the hope, each time, that one can lead an unrestricted life for part of the time. The elation felt while being On stirs even the most inhibited people into a hopeful and lively existence. It is as if the gods breathing fire into a knotted body free it to feel and think, to show expansion and to live with rhythm. Life is then worthwhile and one evades the sure knowledge of a return to an emptiness.

We all carry within us an image of our functioning in an ideal way. This is made up of memories of ourselves and others we may have seen or heard about. The more *real* an experience one gets, the greater the likelihood that we can live with *our* standards, rather than comparing ourselves unfavourably with the ideal.

This process goes into reverse gear when one is afflicted with a deteriorating movement disorder. One is prone to automatically resurrecting the ideal image of oneself and using this illusion to fight off and deny recognition of increasing physical discomfort or immobility. Further, one may increasingly look for treatments aimed at achieving an ideal state rather than to be content with slight benefits. The search for an ultimate drug or the ideal transplant operation, which would do away with supplementary medication, will make one susceptible to miracle-seeking solutions.

Difficulties with dosing may play a central role, manifest in the side effects and the On-Off. It is in the nature of chronic degenerative disorders that a negative reaction to the illness shows itself. The responsive part of the patient takes the drug control of the illness seriously, hoping, as in ordinary illness, that good behaviour will be rewarded. It is a let-down of magical expectation to discover that one is getting worse not better, and more than that, the doctors can't do anything about it.

In sounding out Parkinsonians, they always complain that they are never given enough time to talk to their doctors. In over-booked clinics, discussion with the neurologist is focused on the minutiae of medication rather than the many newly occurring difficulties the patient is experiencing with the condition. A psychotherapeutic listening attitude is not formally installed in training. The patient's working knowledge, as an expert in his disease, needs eventually to surpass that of his doctor if he is to maximize his inner psychological independence. It is surprising how enshrouded in mystery this whole relationship with the doctor, and the need to keep the illness secret, can be. It cuts across class and educational boundaries but predominates in the over-fifties who were too late to benefit in their own upbringing from the liberalization of attitudes in our society.

Revealing one's hopes and frustrations, one's aggressive fantasies and loving wishes, has to it something of the aura of coming out of the closet. Many people, especially the elderly, find this unfamiliar and impossible and therefore withdraw, preferring to rely on their religious belief and personal techniques to shield their feelings.

Treatment of PD demands an alliance of doctor and patient directed to modify and maximize the response of a patient made available by drugs.

Psychotherapy is a valuable, but generally neglected, procedure. In skilled hands, it offers stabilizing insights into the mind-body under the pressure of emotional situations. It is particularly helpful in the depressive reaction to the illness, if not to the underlying depressive core that may be fundamental to it. Finally, it can help with the drug-related depression.

Mobility is naturally affected by fatigue and one soon learns that intermittent rest periods are vital to sustain good On periods. In the early stages of the illness, sleep benefit is such that one wakes up On after a good sleep. Accepting this as part of one's body image in action is important, and self-hatred should not be allowed to interfere with rest. In other words, over-ambitious compensatory efforts may be maintained at a considerable price. One develops a parenting attitude towards one's body if it hasn't developed already. This differs from hypochondriacal attitudes and is much more supportive and understanding. It includes optimizing the time On, keeping one's body in good condition, in expectation of improvements that are awaited in the near future.

The sick body carries with it the penalty of an affected ego, as well as diminishing self-esteem and wounded narcissism; in experiencing a two-part existence in one lifetime, I feel like Lear, who in dotage could say: 'We are not ourselves when nature, being oppressed, commands the mind to suffer with the body'.

CHAPTER 20

Elixir of Life

In reviewing my experiences as an experimental subject for the treatment of PD I naturally question what benefit came of it. Where would I be in the order of things had I accepted the illness and accommodated myself to its natural progression, sat back and gone dutifully to my neurologist twice a year and swallowed the correct dosage of tablets prescribed for me? For one thing, the large number of cells that no longer function would still be in action and unaffected by the experimental procedures.

No matter what the deficit, it wasn't possible for me to accept life as a passive patient. I was driven by my curiosity as a physician to find a way through the illness and motivated by a desire for another chance to lead a dynamic life. To have done it differently, I would have had to have been a different person. I have described my exploration of the origins of my personality and how I faced up to all the losses in my life; my determination fuelled by magical expectations.

Despite the disappointment in the realization that the operation has been of no benefit and has left me facing the continuing degeneration of striatal cells with no resolution at hand, I continue to pursue benefits with the use of new drugs, procedures and improved approaches to the transplant operation.

Oliver Sacks points out there is always a mystery of a magical sort winding through the L-dopa story; that this derives from 'debased metaphysics' and appears as a 'miraculous drug – which will assuage all our hungers and ills and deliver us . . . from our miserable state: metaphorical equivalents of the Elixir of Life'.

In the final analysis, I *am* different now. I am now able to hold back and wait for others to offer themselves for the initial testing, biding my time for a second wave of tests to confirm the potency of the chemical or operation.

Paradoxically, the magic I had sought seems once again around the corner. A research paper published in February 1990 by Prof. Lindvall and others, announced the very best news for a renewal. It describes the successful treatment of a severe Parkinsonian by foetal cell implant. Even though it reports only one case at this time it has been thoroughly documented. With the benefit of a PET scan an increase of dopamine secretion in the affected area is clearly shown.

The response is on the side of the brain opposite to the operation site, showing that this is not a placebo reaction which would show on both sides, nor something produced by a general reaction of the brain to surgical interference.

The ethical problem still delays general adoption of this form of experimentation but the result is a first step to establishing an effective treatment for PD.

The ethical problem of transplantation of tissues may be overcome by the production of fibroblasts (connective tissue cells taken from a scraping of the patient's tissues) genetically engineered to produce levels of dopamine by the insertion of the gene, tyrosine kinase. The advantage of this approach over using foetal cells is that the cells are more accurately defined, are immunologically compatible with the patient and are available as needed. Alternatively, another experiment being prepared for humans is the release of dopamine that has been encapsulated in a plastic polymer which in turn is embedded by operation in the striatum.

Certainly, in the twenty years of my fight against PD, the picture has evolved. What remains to be discovered is the mechanism by which the cell degeneration is initiated and continued. The energy storehouse of the individual cell, the mitochondria, has been implicated and preventive measures and therapeutic strategies may follow. Time and greater activity by researchers is what is called for at the beginning of the 1990s. I hope that this book will act as a spur to hasten the process.

My efforts lent a depth of experience to my life which has given me a greater understanding in my approach to my work and to people. Plummeted into profound despair and regaining hope each time, I have made valuable friends and been in contact with people pursuing the same goals. My life gained a focus; each attempt involved me completely and attracted attention and interest from my friends and family. There was always a promise of success, though each time it was shattered. Most of all, it kept me unfettered by pity and outside the restraint of indifference.

Bibliography

James Parkinson, *Essay on the Shaking Palsy*, London, 1817

Sigmund Freud, *Mourning and Melancholia: The Complete Psychological Works of Sigmund Freud Vol XIV*, London

Oliver Sacks, *Awakenings*, London, 1973. *A Leg To Stand On*, London, 1984

John Bowlby, *Child Care and the Growth of Love*, London, 1953

Anna Freud, *Normality and Pathology in Childhood*, New York, 1965

Donald Calne, *Parkinsonism: Physiology, Pharmacology and Treatment*, London, 1970

Gerald Stern (Editor), *Parkinson's Disease*, London, 1990

David Marsden, Review Article 'Parkinson's Disease' *The Lancet*, 21 April 1990, pages 948–952

Karl Pribram, *Languages of the Brain*, New Jersey, USA, 1971

Joyce McDougall, *Plea for a Measure of Abnormality*, New York, 1980. *Theatres of the Mind*, London 1986. *Theatres of the Body*, London, 1989

Ernest Hartmann, *Functions of Sleep*, Yale University, 1973

Donald Winnicott, *Playing and Reality*, London, 1971

Cecil Todes, 'The child and the dentist: a psychoanalytical view', *British Journal of Medical Psychology* 1972, 45; page 45. 'Inside Parkinsonism ... A Psychiatrist's Personal Experience', *The Lancet* 1983 page 977. 'Idiopathic Parkinson's disease and depression: a psychosomatic view', *Journal of Neurology, Neurosurgery and Psychiatry*, 1984, 47; 298–301

C. Todes, A. Lees, 'The pre-morbid personality of patients

with Parkinson's disease', *Journal of Neurology, Neurosurgery and Psychiatry*, 1985, 48; pages 97–100

W. Birkmayer, P. Riederer, L. Ambrozi and M.B.H. Youdim, 'Implications of combined treatment with Madopar L-deprenyl in Parkinson's disease', *The Lancet*, 1977, pages 439–443

J.P. Frankel, et al., 'Subcutaneous apomorphine in the treatment of Parkinson's disease', *Journal of Neurology Neurosurgery and Psychiatry*, 1990, pages 96–101

E. Hitchcock et al., 'Embryos and Parkinson's disease'. *The Lancet*, 1988, page 1274, Letters to the Editor

J.A. Obeso et al., 'Lisuride infusion pump; a device for the treatment of motor fluctuations in Parkinson's disease', *The Lancet*, 1986, pages 467–470

N. Quinn et al., 'Control of On/Off phenomenon by continuous intravenous infusion of levodopa', *Neurology*, 1984, 34; pages 1131–1136

E-O Backlund et al., 'Transplantation of adrenal medullary tissue to striatum in Parkinsonism; first clinical trials', *Journal of Neurosurgery*, 1985, 62; pages 169–173

O. Lindvall et al., 'Grafts of foetal dopamine neurons survive and improve motor function in PD', *Science*, 1990, 247; pages 574–577.